IT'S **NOT**
BRAIN SURGERY

KRIS A. SMITH, MD

IT'S NOT BRAIN SURGERY

A Neurosurgeon's Prescription
for Health Care Reform

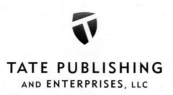

TATE PUBLISHING
AND ENTERPRISES, LLC

Published by Tate Publishing & Enterprises, LLC
127 E. Trade Center Terrace | Mustang, Oklahoma 73064 USA
1.888.361.9473 | www.tatepublishing.com

Tate Publishing is committed to excellence in the publishing industry. The company reflects the philosophy established by the founders, based on Psalm 68:11,
"The Lord gave the word and great was the company of those who published it."

Book design copyright © 2013 by Tate Publishing, LLC. All rights reserved.
Cover design by Rhezette Fiel
Interior design by Deborah Toling

Published in the United States of America

ISBN: 978-1-62746-195-5
1. Medical / Health Policy
2. Business & Economics / Insurance / Health
13.08.06

DEDICATION

To my patients and their families
who have suffered with them.

CONTENTS

INTRODUCTION

What is wrong with American health care? What is good about health care in America? What has caused such an upheaval to lead to the current debate and rhetoric, which fills the newspapers, magazines, and airwaves with passionate arguments from both sides of the political landscape? With the passage of the Affordable Care Act (Obamacare), and the more recent and highly controversial Supreme Court decision to partially uphold Obamacare, there remains anxiety and unrest among physicians, hospital administrators, educators, state governments, politicians, as well as the general public at large. There is no shortage of opinions on the subject as editorial pages and blogs continue to be filled with either outrage or passionate defense of the new law and the Supreme Court decision regarding it. How did we get here? Where are we going? Is Obamacare progress toward increased access and affordability of health care in America, or is it the beginning of the demise of the greatest environment for medical innovation and personalized patient care the world has ever known? The opinions and rhetoric from both sides of the political landscape are so polarizing that it seems impossible to find rational discourse on the subject that is not self-serving for someone's agenda.

As a practicing neurosurgeon, I have been personally interested in not only the practice and science of medicine, but also in the delivery and access to care for my patients. I believe that our current system, or really lack thereof, is badly broken and that reform is desperately needed. The question is not whether reform is needed. It is, how can the system be made to function better with respect to providing access to care, continuing innovation, and improving affordability and doing so without bankrupting the nation?

The current state of health care in America is so complicated with so many implications and ramifications of policy change; it seems that only the human brain itself is more baffling to comprehend. It strikes me, as a neurosurgeon, that we may actually be closer to understanding the complexity of the human brain and the consequences of therapeutic interventions than we are at correctly predicting the results of attempted fixes to the health-care system. In other words, if it were easy to fix, there would be a straightforward solution. I propose that the complexity of the issue requires a much deeper understanding and more thorough research into the problem than can be summarized in a letter to the editor. It takes more than sound bites and catchphrases, which make for easy hits on talk shows.

In trying to understand the brain, we, as a scientific community, attempt to study the history of brain development through evolutionary time as well as the embryology of the nervous system in order to grasp the physiology thereof. This helps us to better understand any therapeutic interventions, which may be recommended. Furthermore, prior to accepting any treatment as standard of care, it must be subjected to experimentation and ideally well-designed clinical trials prior to being generally adopted within the medical community.

I would like to apply a medical metaphor to the current conundrum. America is like a critically ill patient. She is in a recession, diagnosed with encephalopathy (brain dysfunction) in which the brain represents the health-care system. Some other industries, or the government, may envy the position of health care as the brain of America in this analogy, but I could not resist since if we assumed government was the brain, given its inept handling of many issues, the condition would be hopeless, and a "do not resuscitate" (DNR) order would be advised.

The brain represented by the health-care system has some interesting parallels. Health care is projected to soon account for 20 percent of the gross national product (GNP) and the brain, although only weighing about three pounds, or on average 2 percent of the total body weight, receives 20 percent of the blood flow with vital oxygen and glucose (fuel). The central nervous system affects every aspect and organ of the body, similar to how health care affects every single American regardless of age, sex, religion, race, or vocation, be it within the private or public sector. When the brain is sick, the entire body suffers to some degree or another. And severe brain injuries cause complete paralysis of one side of the body or an inability to communicate or see or hear, etc. It may be true that when a patient is brain dead, the heart can continue to pump independently, but what is the point if the patient is comatose? A poor man with his health and vitality is generally much happier than a billionaire in an intensive care unit. A vital organ, such as the heart, can indeed be transplanted to another patient, who can be a very grateful recipient, just like many of our vital manufacturing jobs and industries have been transplanted to other countries due in part to excessive burdens of health-care expenditures for employees of our largest companies. Although entertaining science fiction movies have suggested brain transplantation to be possible, there is really no conceivable way this could be done given our current understanding of the vast complexity and almost infinite number of connections within the brain and between the brain and the rest of our body, which allow us to obtain consciousness and experience the world around us. When the brain is fully functional, it is the organ that provides our greatest joys and accomplishments in creations of art, music, poetry, etc.

Similarly, advances in health care have been heralded as the greatest accomplishments in human history. The accomplishments are so many and so numerous, it is impossible to even fathom the difference in human life today compared someone living one hundred years ago. Small pox has been eradicated from the earth. Polio and leprosy are nearly unknown in advanced countries although still prevalent in the third world. Victims of war injuries in the Civil War and even World War I often died slowly and painfully from infections, and the war injury mortality rate was 40 percent. Now even with the increased lethal power of weapons, our current advanced military hospitals have minimal morbidity and mortality rates. With rehabilitation and advanced prosthetics, some ambitious amputees can now be seen has having an unfair advantage in running races over normal runners. Computer-image guided, minimally invasive techniques have transformed previously untreatable conditions in the brain into routine procedures with good outcomes. We have much work still to do, however, with many conditions, which are as of yet still incurable. Innovations and advancements have indeed been staggering and are a true testament to the great creative power, which has resulted from the freedom of education and scientific exchange afforded in America.

The distribution of health care in America however has not matched the underlying scientific accomplishments. America is now heralded as a military superpower and the leader of the free world; however, our overall health-care statistics lag considerably behind other advanced countries. America's health-care system is in need of resuscitation. Currently, with the passage and gradual implementation of the Affordable Health Care Act commonly referred to as Obamacare, it is undergoing major surgery; however, there is significant disagreement regarding the scope, plan, and extent of the procedure now being employed. Ideally, the treatment should be based on sound scientific evidence in order to make the correct prescription and treatment care plan. I would further propose that health care has been chronically ill and in a state of decline from many years of neglect and abuse leading up to this hospitalization and will need the expertise of multiple specialists over an extended period of rehabilitation, before reaching optimal health.

The goal of intervention must be for an eventually fully functional and sustainable system, which does not result in the demise of the whole patient (America). Thoughtful investigation as to the cause of the problem, such as alcoholism or smoking, which has lead to the buildup of toxins in the brain and lack of blood flow and oxygen will need to be reversed in order for an eventual recovery. Monitoring of brainwaves and appropriate administration of medication and frequent assessments of the brain function, as well as other vital organs, will be necessary for the eventual full recovery. However, notions of radical surgery, such as brain transplantation, are not viable solutions since they would leave the patient permanently disabled or brain dead. Well, enough of the metaphor, you get the picture.

I will attempt to give sufficient background on how we have arrived at our current state of health-care crisis in this country. I will attempt to further inform the reader of many of the problems in the current medical environment, which do not allow for easy solutions. I will ultimately give my personal opinions on how many of these problems may be addressed; however, I do not anticipate it will be simple or painless. It will require some major changes in the philosophy and culture of medicine in America to be successful; however, I do believe it is possible to arrive at a solution with a more rational and a less emotional, and hopefully less political, approach to the problem.

HISTORY OF
AMERICAN HEALTH CARE

In the early 1900s, America began to show its promise as fertile soil for innovation and development in medicine. European medical schools had been long-standing in tradition and clearly had been responsible for substantial progress in many fields; however, reverence for tradition and an inability to question prior thinking and procedures had become stifling for new developments in Europe. Several innovative physicians in America, most notably, Harvey Cushing, the father of modern neurosurgery and also credited for initiating the field of anesthesia and the field of endocrinology, was one of these great innovators. Halstead, Sir William, Osler, the Mayo Brothers, and others began developing new procedures and advanced their respective fields so much that scientists and physicians from Europe began to travel to America to learn from us, rather than the prior state, where, one was not felt to be properly educated, unless one had trained with the European masters.

Beginning with Johns Hopkins University, medical education changed dramatically in the United States compared to all prior settings, here or in Europe. Due to a large philanthropic gift, an institution was established, which was envisioned to incorporate research, outcomes assessment, formal education, and cooperation between medicine and therapeutic surgery. They utilized a gradual hierarchical specialized training of students and residents. Dr. Cushing, as a chief surgical resident under Halstead, flourished in this system by incorporating focused laboratory studies relevant to his clinical experience and became the first recognized specialist in neurosurgery. Cushing popularized the use of ether as a means of providing general anesthesia for his patients and developed the use of monitoring vital signs during the anesthesia to diminish the tendency of mortality by overdose. He was horrified when he went to Europe and witnessed patients who were operated on without any anesthesia, being bound and tied on boards in front of large audiences and succumbed to exhaustion after screaming during their procedures. The field of anesthesia still utilizes similar anesthetic records of vital sign documentation during surgical procedures today.

Harvard, Yale, the University of Chicago, and others adopted the Hopkins Model and became respected around the world as leaders in medical innovation and medical education. The Mayo brothers developed a private institution in a cornfield in Minnesota, which became famous because of the surgical technique and positive outcomes obtained there, due to the surgical skills and adaptations of sterile techniques and anesthesia. There arose medical associations and societies, which fostered education and sharing of techniques and therapeutic theories. Journals became established as the medium to portray new insights and knowledge to be adapted and adopted by others. Intense, but mostly healthy, competition between physicians arose regarding getting credit for the latest innovation or medical discovery. Lavish meetings were held during which data and theories were presented to be accepted, or refuted, by professional peers. Disagreements and competition between Cushing and Dandy (initially his resident, and later his greatest competitor) were legendary at some of these early medical meetings attended by thousands of physicians. With time, America clearly became the leader in medical innovation, and Europeans came here to learn of the new medical techniques developed and perfected within the innovative American system.

Well-trained American physicians could hang up their shingles with pride, knowing they had received the best training with the latest innovations in the world. America as a country was booming with new immigrants arriving by hoards to the land of opportunity. Business and industry flourished with nearly unrestrained capitalism. Railways connected the vast country between the East and West coasts. Physicians were well respected and sought after in large and small communities alike. Treatments were relatively simple, and often meager, or ineffective, by today's standards. Payments to physicians were given directly by the patient, or family, and were quite modest. Bartering of goods for services by the physician was relatively common in small towns. Meals for house calls were common practice, etc. Even Harvey Cushing in his early days would perform surgery in the kitchen of the home of the patient because the operating room environment was not much different.

The majority of patients treated in the developing training hospital settings like Hopkins were charity cases. The patients were desperate, many died, autopsies were performed on most, and medical knowledge was gained. The training physicians received meager salaries and worked nearly like slaves for their superiors. Wealthy patients were treated in private clinics or in separate wards of the hospitals and were charged sometimes incredibly excessive fees. A charge of $10,000 by Halstead for surgery was common for the wealthiest patients, which in today's dollars would be about $300,000.

As treatments became more complicated, however, the need for transportation of patients with complex problems to specialized centers began. The percentage of patients treated in larger specialty centers was miniscule compared to today and depended highly upon the sophistication of the local physician and his personal connections and the means of the family. People understood that they were completely responsible for their own health and for any payment to restore good health if possible.

My grandmother on my mother's side, for example, fell under a train at age eight and had both lower legs amputated in this tragic accident. This was in 1914, prior to antibiotics and sterile surgical technique. She ultimately underwent eleven revisions and wound debridements of her amputated limbs. Looking back on this time, it was miraculous that she survived. She never talked of it bitterly but described being pulled around for years in a little wagon prior to being able to have prosthetic limbs made. Her family traveled along the railroad lines in the western United States and Canada, never really being seen at a major medical center. She described to me how rudimentary her first prosthetic limbs were and how, over years, multiple improvements were made with each new set. There were no government agencies or third-party payers. Her family was by no means wealthy, as her father was a construction worker and prospector, but somehow could afford her medical expenses. I am sure the expenses were somewhat burdensome to the family, but they were paid because they could be, and had to be; and there was no alternative solution, other than going without limbs or fixing them in the wood shop behind the house. The price of the procedures and the artificial limbs reflected their real value and not a trumped-up charge to a third-party payer justified by medical liability coverage. She was notoriously independent and strong willed and became educated as a school teacher, becoming one of the first school teachers in Las Vegas, Nevada, when the population of Las Vegas was only two thousand people. She roamed the barren roads of the desert southwest alone in her model A Ford prior to meeting and marrying my grandfather. On a personal side note, she was truly one of my greatest inspirations to go into medicine in the first place.

As unbelievable as it may sound, my father's mother also had a tragic accident at age three. She was run over by a hay combine driven by her father on their farm in Washington State, which amputated both of her lower legs below the knees as well. Her family described the horrific scene to me of her father's hands needing to be pried from her bleeding stumps by the medical personnel. She also underwent many revisions and eventually received prosthetic limbs. I grew up believing that all grandmothers came with removable wooden legs that they took off at night before going to bed. Later as a college/medical student, I accompanied my grandmothers occasionally on visits to doctor's offices and to prosthetists. I remember viewing spinal X-rays, which, as the orthopedist explained to me, showed the degenerative changes resulting from years of a compensatory altered gait.

I share this background for two reasons: first, to reveal how different medicine was less than a century ago, but also to give insight into myself as a physician. I don't think of myself as unique in having had profound influences, which drove me to choose this career. I am being honest with myself and with you as the reader in stating that this was not primarily a financially motivated decision. Sure, in the back of my mind, I knew that doctors were supposed to make a decent living, but it was not about becoming rich. It is about a love of science and biology and a desire to help others. Not cold science without application, but personally fulfilling application of science for the alleviation of pain and suffering and for the betterment of humanity on a one patient at a time basis.

I see the same youthful enthusiasm in the residents I help to train and in the medical students who rotate through our neurosurgical service. We have numerous weekly conferences and research meetings, all of which are completely and solely about the advancement of the understanding of disease processes and how better to address them for our patients. It is intellectually stimulating, unbelievably complex and challenging, and humbling all at the same time. It is deeply rewarding when you actually make a difference in patient's lives and an often unspoken bond develops between the patient, family, and treating physician. Thank you notes, special small gifts, baked goods, etc., have touched me deeply from numerous grateful patients and families. Especially touching are cards from families whose loved ones died in spite of all we could do. These are not just words, and I am not alone among my colleagues who share the same sentiments in saying that "*It is a profound privilege to be a physician!*" We share in these emotional and trying challenges that our patients face, and fortunately in 2013, we often have at our disposal meaningful interventions, which can alleviate pain and suffering, and even sometimes cure them of disease processes, which would have been hopeless less than a hundred years ago.

HISTORY OF HEALTH INSURANCE IN AMERICA

Blue Cross was the first American health insurance company. It was developed initially by Justin Ford Kimball in 1929 at Baylor University in Texas. It was first designed for teachers to be able to afford hospital care. The fee was $6 per year to cover up to twenty-one days of hospital care at Baylor. The plan was so successful that it was adopted by other employee groups and hospitals throughout the country. The American Hospital Association (AHA) eventually adopted the Blue Cross symbol for insurance plans, which met certain standards of coverage for the majority of hospitals nationally. Blue Shields was developed ten years later in 1939 for the lumberyard workers and mining camps in the Pacific Northwest. Monthly payments were made by employers for their workers to medical service bureaus, which were comprised of affiliated groups of physicians who agreed to treat the employees at contracted rates.

Thus began the concept and practice of employee health benefits. Workers in these somewhat dangerous professions would have clearly preferred to work for an employer who offered such medical coverage compared to accepting the risk himself. Eventually, these practices became widely adopted by major employers for virtually all vocations throughout the country. Initially, there were major tax breaks for employers offering these benefits as they were regarded as social welfare plans and were tax exempt. Blue Cross and Blue Shields eventually merged resulting in combined coverage for hospitals and physicians.

In 1986, however, the tax reform act was passed to revoke the tax exempt status because the insurance plans were often commercial entities and made substantial profits. Today there are numerous different agencies of Blue Cross/Blue Shield, which function as independent franchises under the global heading. Most are defined by state boundaries; however, the largest ones involve multiple states. Some are for profit and others are not-for-profit. Some are investor-owned, publically traded companies and others are not.

It is impossible to overstate the effect that insurance has had on the delivery and practice of health care in America. As procedures have become more complicated, expensive, and hospital based, insurance has eased the burden of these high costs for patients and families who needed care. The concept that most people fail to recognize however is the effect of separating the cost of insurance and health care away from the individual and toward the employer. This separation has caused the illusion to the patient that health care is essentially free to them and that their employer is responsible for the payment of their care. This is painfully apparent when talking to patients today. When a test or procedure is mentioned, they typically ask, "Is it covered by my insurance?" If the answer is yes, then no hesitation exists regarding the test or procedure in question, no matter what the actual cost may be. The discussion ends without any question of the necessity or the test or the possibility of less expensive alternatives. Patients seem to think of insurance as a blank check for them to spend without any real consequences of cost for their personal health-care decisions.

To make matters worse, as regards to the cost of medicine, physicians have no incentive to not order more tests or procedures either. Doctors sometimes in fact have significant monetary incentives to order anything that may be even remotely indicated, especially if they actually own the laboratory or X-ray machines and can charge for their use. The 1960s and '70s were considered by doctors to be the heyday of medicine since there were minimal regulations or cost-control mechanisms. Most patients had insurance, and when bills were submitted to the insurance companies, they were paid without questions or additional forms or codes to be submitted. Physicians became very successful small businessmen. They invested in themselves by purchasing office buildings and laboratory and X-ray equipment. Some had local pharmacies in their own office buildings, so if a prescription were filled, they could earn money on that aspect of care as well. Pharmaceutical companies catered to doctors and appealed to all incentives to promote their specific medications. Hospitals catered to physicians as well because if the doctor admitted a patient to their facility, money was earned. Better yet, if a surgical procedure was performed, then significant fees could be charged to the private insurance companies. Because there was a complete disconnect between the patient charges and the party responsible for the payment, there were essentially no market forces in place to put a check into the process of cost escalation. And escalate the costs did!

There has never been a time when everyone carried private insurance. Those who were self-employed or who worked for small companies, which did not provide insurance, were at a significant disadvantage and had high out-of-pocket expenses. It was commonly accepted that there existed enough slush from the private insurance billing to more than compensate for those who had no means to pay; although bill collectors would still go after all they could and had the legal means to do so. The biggest problem however arose with the elderly who were no longer working and had no prospects of employer-based benefits.

The idea of government-based health insurance actually began in the early 1900s primarily at the state level. There was strong interest in providing for health coverage for the military around World War I; however, there was significant disagreement after the war. Initially, the labor unions opposed government insurance and felt threatened by it. The American Medical Association (AMA) and the American Hospital Association (AHA) voted that they were unequivocally opposed to government-financed health care in 1920. The private insurance industry was most vociferously opposed to the idea and lobbied strongly against any public health insurance program. The mood of the public began to shift strongly toward government assistance in health care after the Great Depression of the 1930s.

Prior to the Depression, the individualistic and capitalistic ideals were strongly in place, especially in the minds of physicians, who prided themselves on ingenuity and independence. Physicians opposed public intervention into any part of the practice of medicine. However, the hopelessness of the Depression allowed the public mind-set to shift dramatically toward a more collective thought process and more socialistic ideals. The "New Deal" of President Roosevelt encompassed multiple government-run programs aimed at solving social issues and combating massive unemployment. The most notable new program signed into law was the Social Security Act.

Government based health insurance was in reality thought to be included in these programs from the beginning as part of the Social Security Act. There was however strong opposition to the healthcare component by the medical profession among others and a compromise was reached to pursue the employment insurance component as the main thrust of the new legislation. Of note, the father-in-law of President Roosevelt's son James was none other than the before mentioned neurosurgeon Harvey Cushing. Dr. Cushing, as well as the president's personal physicians, likely had significant influence on this matter and warned of the possibility of losing the entire legislation if they tried to ram the public health insurance down the doctors' throats. The health insurance program was completely dropped from the Social Security Act when it was signed into law in 1935.

President Roosevelt clearly wanted to have national health insurance on the legislative docket in 1938 and 1939, and there was significant public support for many aspects of his plan, except he was politically vulnerable, due to continued unemployment and a recession at the time. AMA opposition was also quite strong. All hopes of passage failed with the onset of World War II after Poland was invaded in 1939.

After World War II, employer-based health insurance became fully established as the primary means of insurance coverage for most Americans. Companies received tax incentives and deductions for providing health insurance to their employees. Benefits packages became and certainly remain a vital aspect of the company's ability to attract and maintain quality employees. Multiple different options of insurance plans began to emerge with alphabet soup labels such as PPOs (preferred provider organizations) and HMOs (health maintenance organizations).

HMOs developed primarily as a means to contain costs but promoted a concept and philosophy of prepaid health care. They made promises to patients to cover routine physicals and preventative screening tests in hopes of avoiding emergency room visits and catching problems early. Incentives were placed to prevent referrals to specialists because that is where most of the high costs were generated. People would sign up for these new insurance products with the name insurance purposefully deleted in the branding of the product. The goals and ideas of health maintenance are certainly worthy. Supposedly, preventive medicine would be encouraged and diseases would be detected earlier, resulting in less need for later and more expensive salvage treatments like surgery. Routine office visit required decreased expenses and minimal co-pays. This could and probably does have the effect of promoting more visits to the primary care physicians and in the field of pediatrics. Increased utilization of vaccinations and some truly beneficial preventative measures are realized. However, the shift of the perception of responsibility for one's health and the payment for one's health services was clearly shifted away from the individual and toward the provider of the health insurance (HMO) company.

What many people did not realize is that the primary care physician (PCP) in an HMO was placed in a position of gatekeeper for more expensive tests and procedures and had financial incentives to not order these tests or to consult specialists. It would literally come out of the PCPs back pocket if a test or consultation were ordered. This reverse incentive actually sets up an adversarial relationship between PCPs and specialists rather than a mutually beneficial one. Traditionally, PCPs foster relationships with specialists who treat their patients well because they feel responsible to have the patients that they care for, and feel personally responsible for, to have the best care. The patients, if pleased with the care they received, are generally grateful for being referred to a good specialist and appreciate the fact that their trusted PCP knew enough to send him or her to someone who was both caring and qualified. The specialist who received the referral also attempts to foster the relationship with the PCP because he knows that if the patient does well and is pleased with the care provided and gives positive feedback to the referring PCP, that PCP is likely to refer additional patients in the future. That has been the means for decades of building a successful specialty practice.

What was so wrong with the symbiotic relationship between PCPs and specialists? Cynics would say there are potential abuses or kickbacks to be gained from this system, which could artificially increase unnecessary referrals and promotes cost increases. I have never personally seen or even heard of specific examples of gross financial kickbacks between specialists and PCPs; however, I do not doubt that in unusual or extreme cases, they have occurred. I certainly have seen minimal examples, which could be construed by a cynic as an example of a kickback, like sending a PCP a Christmas food basket and thank you card. I also learned as a medical student that in small towns, general surgeons would often allow PCPs to scrub in on surgical cases as a first assistant and the PCP would be able to bill for these assistant fees. The PCP could be persuaded to refer preferentially to surgeons who allowed this to occur as opposed to surgeons who typically have their partners or hired physician assistants to provide this service. A supercynic might even suggest that an unscrupulous PCP might even refer a patient for unnecessary surgery in order to collect these surgical assistant fees. Has this ever happened in the history of medicine? Probably. But is this a common problem of cost escalation? I really don't think so.

One may doubt the validity of medical ethics and the honor of physicians in today's society. But in my experience, the code of ethics and degree of honor of the vast majority of physicians is alive and well. Almost all physicians I personally know take great pride in their responsibility of taking care of patients and having their patient's best interests at heart. In other words, the honorable physician is the rule rather than the exception. But physicians are not perfect, and they certainly are influenced by financial incentives.

In a traditional private practice, physicians are small business owners and are certainly concerned about ways to improve the financial viability and success of their practice. In simplest terms, successful doctors build a practice by being good doctors. When they treat patients well and compassionately, they gain a favorable reputation, word of mouth spreads quickly, and the practice builds with time. As with all businesses, however, the physician looks at how he spends his time and what is most cost-effective and efficient. Consciously, or subconsciously, the doctor analyzes and balances the time he spends with individual patients to be caring and thorough against how much time he can afford to spend with each patient since he is really not paid by the hour but rather by patient encounter. No doctor can afford to spend three hours with one patient if the encounter is billed at $100. Likewise, no patient is going to feel good about a five-minute, rushed assessment of a complex problem by his doctor and finding out that he was compensated several hundred dollars for such an interaction. It is a constant balance between efficiency, compassion, completeness, and clinical accuracy. The most important asset a doctor possesses is his reputation among his patients and his peers.

So let's go back to the point of HMO disincentives. The goal of the HMO board of directors and CEOs is to curtail costs. When the PCP no longer receives compensation for each patient encounter but rather a prepayment for the number of patients he is caring for, there has been a complete shift in the doctor-patient relationship and contract. In the HMO model, the PCPs as gatekeepers literally receive a kickback bonus directly related to the number of tests and referrals they do *not* order. By some standardized quotas and goals and bell-shaped curves, a typical number of tests/referrals per patient life years is set. The doctor is financially penalized by exceeding these norms and rewarded if his monthly or yearly numbers of tests/referrals are below the other doctors in his HMO group. If the doctor is an owner/stockholder in the HMO group, his financial incentive is then not so much dependent on his reputation as a physician but rather is dependent on his efficiency and frugality within the HMO system or company. Is that the incentive that you want your PCP to have? What are the consequences of this paradigm shift in the doctor-patient relationship?

The HMO assumption is that smaller co-pays and shifting visits from specialists to PCPs saves money and prevents diseases or detects them earlier by more routine physical exams and preventative health care visits. Is this assumption true? As in all complex issues, it is probably true in some sense and in some circumstances but certainly not in all circumstances and not for every patient condition or disease. Certainly *if* doctors could positively influence patients to loose weight, change their diet, stop smoking, limit alcohol and drug use and unprotected sexual promiscuity, there would likely be an actual measurable decline in overall health care needs of many patients by reducing early strokes and heart attacks and AIDs and diabetes, etc.

We physicians only wish we had this kind of influence on our patient's lives. Maybe there are some patients who actually heed the advice of their doctor and make meaningful lifestyle changes, but in all reality, these patients are the minority. Societal trends and cultural shifts and pressures are much more influential on teenagers and young adults than any brief visit with even the most charismatic doctor. Middle-aged people who have now gained a sense of their own mortality often do seek out health advice as part of a midlife crisis. Speaking from personal experience, they may alter diets and begin running marathons or join a gym in hopes of cheating the grim reaper for as long as possible. But does that have anything to do with a doctor encounter and the need for tests or procedures?

I propose that disease happens! Some diseases are preventable and some are not. If a disease process is happening in your body, you unfortunately don't have control over that process until it is detected. Much of your tendency to develop a disease process can be blamed on your parents. Not that they were abusive, but they simply imported to you the genetic material that makes you who you are. Someday, we may be able to alter genes and gene expression, but at this time, we are simply becoming more and more aware of how important a person's genetic material is in imparting susceptibility to disease or the lack thereof. Hopefully you are still with me, but I'll now get back to the point of the HMO issue.

If a person has a symptom, which is due to an adverse process occurring in the body, ignoring that symptom, and simply hoping that it goes away on its own, only works if the body can heal itself. The body's amazing immune system truly has adapted over eons of time to allow us to survive many infections and injuries. However, in all times prior to ours, people often died prematurely of many disease processes. Sadly, prior to the year 1900, approximately half of all children died prior to reaching the age of five years, most often due to infections. It has been the advent of modern medicine, which has allowed us to detect these processes and alter the natural history in a favorable way for many patients. Therefore, by ordering tests and performing these medically proven procedures before the symptoms have progressed too far is imperative in order to have the best long-term outcome for that patient.

As a medical student, resident, and attending physician, I have encountered many patients who had initially presented to a PCP with neurological symptoms secondary to an adverse process in the brain or spine, which was dismissed, not just initially, but repeatedly prior to ordering the appropriate test or referral. I am not stating this to be unfairly critical of PCPs. It is easy for me to see a patient after an MRI is ordered and the diagnosis has been made to apply the "retrospec-toscope" and easily associate the presenting signs and symptoms to the problem, which is now obvious. It is a far different thing to solve the puzzle initially and play detective with obscure clues from sometimes elusive patient-historians. Nevertheless, the point is that by denying the existence of a disease process and avoiding the early detection of it only compounds the problem and makes the necessary intervention much more difficult and usually much more expensive as well in the long run. Also, the patient may suffer significantly during this time of delay and denial.

One illustrative patient comes to mind. A middle-aged female patient of mine originally presented to her PCP with episodic complaints of severe anxiety. These episodes were also associated with lapses in memory and poor work performance. The episodes had been building in both severity and frequency for several months prior to seeking out medical attention. Her PCP ascribed the adverse events to stress although no clear changes in life stressors were identified. No tests were ordered and antianxiety medications were prescribed. Initially, the medicine appeared to work; however, the events became refractory to increasing doses of medication and additional medications were prescribed until she was on a combination of four medications without controlling the anxiety.

Psychological counseling was performed over years of time but had no effect at alleviating the episodes. She also was suffering from significant side effects from the multiple medications. Ultimately after many years, an astute psychiatrist felt that the episodes were atypical for stress-related anxiety and referred the patient to a neurologist, who in turn ordered an MRI. The MRI showed an unusual abnormality in the brain involving the insula and amygdala. After additional time and a follow-up MRI examination, it was determined that the discovered abnormality was implicated as a possible cause of her anxiety by means of focal seizure activity. I recommended an operation and, after much additional discussion, surgically removed it, in spite of it being in a relatively difficult location. Fortunately, after this procedure, the episodes resolved and she was ultimately weaned off all but one of her medications and has resumed an essentially normal life. She, however, suffered from these paralyzing fearful episodes for years unnecessarily due to a lack of appropriate tests and referrals. I could cite numerous other examples of brain tumors, which had progressed to enormous sizes by the time an appropriate test or referral was made in spite of symptom onset at a much earlier time.

The point that I am making is simply that you do not want to be enrolled in an insurance system, which is based on a negative incentive regarding the early diagnosis of a medical problem. If you have a truly significant medical problem that is not self-limiting, you would like to know about it sooner than later. In an HMO model, where the payments are all collected up front and the doctor keeps a piece of the pie for not ordering tests, it is financially preferable for you to never be diagnosed until it is too late. Hospice care is much less expensive than years of extended life, which might include multiple surgeries, radiation, chemo-therapy, and frequent surveillance imaging from the HMO's stockholder's point of view. In a fee-for-service model, it is still costly to your insurance company if you are diagnosed early and receive expensive treatments, but at least your greatest advocate to stay alive, your doctor, is not consciously or subconsciously conflicted financially in his role as your health care provider.

I am certain that I have just offended many competent and compassionate physicians employed in HMOs. That was not my intent. I could again refer back to my earlier point of generally high medical ethics among physicians and certainly HMO-employed physicians are not exempt from this claim. I am sure most are very good doctors and function very well for their patients in their system. I am simply stating that financial incentives may play an adversarial role even on an unconscious level, just like excessive tests may be ordered with financially incentivized physicians, who are part owners of an imaging center in a fee-for-service model.

Accountable care organizations (ACOs) are a vital part of Obamacare and are part of an attempt at cost containment. The concept of ACOs appears very similar to HMOs in my opinion. The hospital that I work in has now become part of an accepted ACO. As I understand it, an ACO receives funds from the government for the responsibility of a certain number of patient lives. Costs utilized to treat these patients are deducted from a promised prepaid cost to maintain health for these people. Therefore, the financial incentives are to decrease procedures and tests for these patients rather than to charge for the services as in a fee-for-service model. Again, I have serious reservations regarding the philosophy of this concept and fear that it produces a deleterious effect on the doctor-patient relationship. I have heard discussions among hospital administrators sounding quite confused about how this is supposed to work. I have heard statements like, "All this time we have been focusing on providing equipment and facilities for procedures to be done and for efficiently performing those procedures for patients, and now we're supposed to avoid using all of this equipment in order to make more money instead of gaining money by performing these procedures with this equipment."

Today there are very complicated negotiations between hospital and physician groups and insurance companies regarding insurance coverage and compensation for services rendered. Most physician groups operate on percentages of compensation which are based on the Medicare rates. Therefore Medicare rates are vitally important for determining physician incomes and the availability of certain treatments. There is a complicated coding system called the ICD-9 system, which determines a basic level of compensation for most procedures. If some procedures do not have an appropriately assigned ICD-9 code, the government and most insurance companies will not cover the procedure. It has been a very frustrating experience for some of my patients who have very rare diseases with known treatments but which are unapproved or labeled "experimental." These treatments simply cannot be performed because the hospital will not admit the patient without preapproval for payment. Some complicated procedures have multiple add-on codes, which increase the reimbursement and are attempts at recognizing that some cases are more difficult than others. There has been much criticism for some physicians in their inappropriate and excessive use of additional codes in order to increase their reimbursement rates.

Several years ago, there was a significant fallout from some less-than-ethical physicians who practiced a coding tactic known as unbundling in which multiple small codes were added on or billed as individual procedures in order to increase their reimbursement. There remains a certain prevalence of Medicare fraud with excessive charges and there are very stiff penalties for physicians found guilty of such financial abuses of the system. I am personally aware of single spine operations with physician bills in excess of $100,000. This is absolutely unconscionable. How could a physician look a patient in the eye and knowingly charge that patient more than most people's annual income for a single day's work? Not to excuse these physicians, but they are not looking the patients in the eyes. They are charging a deep-pocket insurance company, who they feel have blank checkbooks. This is an example of disconnection between the traditional doctor-patient relationship of the past.

Larger group practices negotiate with insurance companies regarding the reimbursement rates for their services. It is interesting to note that physicians are prohibited from discussing their surgical charges with other competing physicians. Typically rates are based on a percentage of Medicare reimbursements, and usually the reimbursement rates of insurance companies are higher by factors of 1.2–2.5 times the Medicare rates. Sometimes there are significant sticking points on both sides of the negotiations and occasionally no agreement can be reached and patients covered under these insurance plans may not be seen or operated on by physicians in these groups without a contract. This is a very difficult dynamic for the patient because the patient has no voice in these negotiations and usually does not have any knowledge of what is at stake for them personally. There are surprisingly different skill and experience levels between physicians of different groups and in different locations. Obviously the scenario is not ideal for the patients because the patient's right to choose the physician of their choice has been undercut, without any say in the matter, and with possible significant consequences to their health care and their very lives.

It should be noted that there are severe problems with many of the current codes and the low level of reimbursement, which have been achieved over the last several years of cost cutting. For example, the code reimbursement rate for an appendectomy by a general surgeon is only $300. Although this is not a complicated or typically difficult procedure, this amount of money is in no way commensurate to the level training and time required for the procedure. Prior to performing the procedure, the general surgeon must take a history from the patient, examine the patient, and evaluate all of the labs and diagnostic procedures and many times order and interpret additional X-rays or CT or ultrasound scans to make an appropriate diagnosis and then discuss with the patient the risks and alternatives to surgical removal of the appendix. Furthermore, the $300 reimbursement is a three-month all-inclusive fee, including all postoperative care and office visits for three months.

No general surgeon can possibly afford to maintain a practice and pay his office staff and nurses with these levels of reimbursement, not to mention taxes to be paid. Nothing against plumbers, but most people pay more for a typical service call by a plumber in the middle of the day compared to this fee for a general surgeon to save a life in the middle of the night. I am personally very grateful to a general surgeon for operating on me before my appendix ruptured on New Year's Eve when I was only eight years old. I was told of a mini celebration in the operating room over my tiny anesthetized body at the stroke of midnight when they pulled out my appendix only hours before it should have ruptured.

I have seen hospital bills from some of my patients as well as from hospital charges from admissions of my own family members. The numbers are staggering. Sticker shock doesn't even come close to describing these seemingly ridiculous charges from the hospital. I am aware of certain charges for equipment and supplies from surgical procedures. It seems absurd to me that a disposable instrument used for only an hour on one patient can have a charge in excess of $2,000. Single rods or screws and plates for spine stabilization have costs in the thousands of dollars. A rechargeable internal pulse generator has a charge of $28,000. There is no way that manufacturing, marketing, and distribution costs justify these charges.

It is certainly a relief to note that the insurance companies have contracted for rates that are much more reasonable and that the hospital has agreed to accept the insurance payments as payment-in-full most of the time. The question becomes what happens to the accounting of all of that money that is never paid? Does anyone get stuck with the full charge payment? Unfortunately, if someone does not have insurance, the hospital can go after an individual for the full price. With hospital bills in excess of hundreds of thousands of dollars, the only recourse for most patients is to file for bankruptcy. Obviously this helps no one. The individual is labeled as having bad credit, and the hospital must eat the cost and lose the money spent on those procedures and devices. It is likely that the hospital feels justified in charging excessively high fees in order to attempt to recoup money from these continued losses. This is another example of a vicious cycle of ridiculousness in medical economics. The charges are more like Monopoly money than real dollars. That is of course unless you're stuck without insurance and end up being responsible for those trumped-up charges. It seems unlikely that traditional market forces can be optimized and utilized in the medical system unless realistic real dollar values and transparent accounting systems are in play.

MEDICARE

I have already discussed Medicare in the previous chapter somewhat tangentially; however, I will attempt to summarize the problems associated with this program more directly in this chapter.

President Harry Truman attempted to establish a national health insurance plan in 1945, but there was significant resistance with private insurance groups and the established medical community regarding the dangers of socialized medicine. By the end of his term, the focus had shifted to developing a national program of health coverage for Social Security beneficiaries. It was not until July 30, 1965, that Medicare and its companion program Medicaid were signed into law by President Lyndon Johnson as part of his "Great Society." Ex-President Truman was the first to enroll in Medicare, and all citizens over age sixty-five were eligible, and the initial number was around nine million people who were covered in this new plan. In 1972, President Nixon signed his Social Security Amendments, which established that persons under age sixty-five with permanent disabilities and specifically those with end-stage renal disease requiring dialysis were covered under this program so that by the end of 1972, there were 20.4 million Medicare beneficiaries. People who were disabled and poor and receiving supplementary Social Security income were automatically eligible for Medicaid. The Health Care Finance Administration (HFCA) was established under the Department of Health Education and Welfare in 1977 to administer the Medicare and Medicaid programs. Approximately 1,500 Federal employees were transferred from the social security administration to the HFCA at its inception.

HMO payments were authorized in 1972 as well as some expanded services including chiropractic care, speech and physical therapy, and hospice benefits were temporarily added in 1982 and permanently included in 1986. The system of diagnostic related groups (DRGs) was implemented in 1983, and most Federal civilian employees also became eligible for coverage in this year. In 1985, COBRA (Consolidated Omnibus Reconciliation Act) was enacted to make all new government employees automatically eligible for Medicare. And EMTALA (Emergency Medical Treatment and Labor Act) was added as a stipulation for all institutions with emergency rooms accepting Medicare payments to be required to provide emergency and stabilizing treatments for all individuals, regardless of insurance or legal citizenship status.

Prescription drugs and catastrophic illnesses were initially covered in 1988; however, this was repealed only one year later in 1989. A payment fee schedule for physician services was implemented in 1992. The Medicare + Choice component was included in the

Balanced Budget Act of 1997 to attempt to curtail the rising cost of the Medicare program and then further refined due to funding restrictions in 1999. The Benefits Improvement and Protection Act of 2000 increased Medicare payments to providers and Medicare + Choice plans and reduced certain Medicare beneficiary co-payments and began covering some preventative services. Initially in 1965, the Medicare part B coverage premium for physician payments was $3 per month but had increased to $54 per month by the year 2000 and the total number of Medicare recipients had increased to forty million people.

In 2001, the secretary of Health and Human Services, Tommy Thompson, renamed the HFCA the Centers for Medicare and Medicaid Services (CMS). The total Medicare spending in 2001 was $217 billion. The Medicare Prescription Drug, Improvement and Modernization Act of 2003 was signed into law in 2003 by President Bush with outpatient prescription drug benefit coverage under Medicare beginning in 2006. Medicare + Choice was renamed the Medicare Advantage program in 2007 with financial incentives for private health plans to contract with Medicare and established a new way of assessing Medicare financial status by looking at the general revenues as a percentage of total Medicare spending.

Beginning in 2007, Medicare beneficiaries with individual incomes more than $80,000 per year were required to pay a higher monthly premium based on their modified adjusted gross income. The medical Board of Trustees calculated that general revenue will exceed 45 percent of Medicare funding within the succeeding seven years triggering a "Medicare funding warning." An extension act was passed to prevent a required 10 percent reduction in Medicare physician payments and allowed for a 0.5 percent increase for physician payments through June of 2008. Each year since this vote, an extension has been passed, called the "doc fix," but the prospect of a cut causes tremendous angst among physicians each time the vote comes up. The current legally required cut to physicians is 24 percent, but it is anticipated that continued votes for deferments of these cuts will continue to be passed, but there is no guarantee.

Initially there were about eight to ten working individuals for every person on Medicare. Currently, that ratio has dropped to 3.7:1 and, unless changes are enacted, the ratio will be less than 2:1 in 2030 when all baby boomers will have reached the age of eligibility. The initial cost of Medicare far exceeded the initial estimates, and it has been widely speculated that President Johnson purposefully understated the projected costs to get the program passed in the legislature. The program was projected to cost $9 billion annually by 1990, but the actual cost in 1990 was $67 billion, and the most recent numbers from 2010 were around $500 billion. Currently 15 percent of the entire national budget is spent on this program. It has been concluded that if Congress had any idea in 1965 that the Medicare program would have grown to this size and scope, they never would have passed it.

The other very complicated aspect of Medicare is that it does not function like a public government program in other countries. The administration of the medical care, including the contracting with doctors and hospitals and the processing of the billing and the collection of funds are administered through private insurance companies and HMOs. At Medicare's inception in 1965, there were over one hundred separate insurance companies, which administered the care. Each of these companies had different forms and variations in protocols and levels of administrative bureaucracy. Over time, there have been numerous measures taken to consolidate and simplify the technicalities of health-care administration and the process has resulted in thinning the herd down to thirty-eight present companies. Many have suggested that a single government payer system with a single mechanism of administration would be more efficient. I really do not know if this is true; however, it seems that extra layers of middlemen between the payer source (the government) and the health-care providers (the doctors and hospitals) add additional costs and complexity to the system.

One thing I do know is that it is extremely frustrating to have a patient referred to me for specialty care, which I am more than willing to provide, and to be denied the opportunity to care for that patient by a secondary insurance company when the source of the funds for that patient is Medicare or Medicaid, the same source that provides for the care of other patients with the same condition on a routine basis but is administered by other companies. My office last week had to spend an entire day attempting to appease an angry family and their referring neurologist regarding an unfortunate patient with epilepsy who has been trying to get an office appointment with me for four months unsuccessfully. She is an excellent candidate for potentially curative surgery but has been denied access to my care by the insurance company who is the administrator of the Medicaid plan. The administrators of these plans take money off the top from the state and federal government for the promise of providing care for these patients, but then deny the care when it is needed and then leave us to deal with the angry patients because of it. It is very hard for me to believe that this is the best way to administer medicine in this country.

OBAMACARE

The Patient Protection and Affordable Care Act (PPACA), commonly referred to as Obamacare, represents a massive undertaking from the federal government to address the health-care problem in America. The goal of Obamacare is to decrease the number of uninsured individuals within the country and that is certainly admirable. Believe me when I say that all physicians would love to have far less uninsured patients to take care of for free. So then why are so many physicians opposed to Obamacare?

I must confess that I have not read the over-two-thousand pages, similar to most of the legislators who voted to pass it. But I have read several nonpartisan reviews and summaries of the bill. My main concern regarding Obamacare is that it does not address the underlying causes of price escalation and does nothing to address the issue of malpractice-induced defensive medicine. It is also concerning that there are reported to be twenty-one additional taxes to be imposed on the American public and countless additional agencies and regulatory stipulations included within the PPACA. It strikes me as counterintuitive that some of these taxes to support Obamacare actually come from the pro-

viders of health insurance and medical devices. There
is an excise tax of 40 percent on insurance premiums
over ten thousand dollars, and a sixty-billion-dollar fee
on health insurance providers. There is also a twenty-
seven-billion dollar fee for branded drug manufacturers
and a twenty-billion-dollar tax on medical devices. If
you increase the taxes on medical devices, drugs and
private insurance, doesn't that indirectly increase the
costs of medicine to the public because these increases
in costs will be passed on to the consumer? Furthermore,
it is estimated that there will still be twenty-five million uninsured people after the program is fully implemented by the year 2019.

I believe I am accurate in stating that most physicians are very nervous about the implications and ramifications of Obamacare as it gradually becomes implemented. Generally stated, additional regulations and
administrative bureaucratic controls have never made
the lives of physicians or their patients easier. I have
major concerns with appointed officials deciding which
care is available for which patient. I do not believe that
the Accountable Care Organization (ACO) model,
similar to the HMO idea, is a valid mechanism for
controlling costs and providing compassionate and
efficient care. It is also concerning that health saving
accounts, which in my opinion have an excellent ability of making insurance more affordable and applying
market pressures for cost controls, are specifically eliminated in Obamacare. And also diminishing Medicare
in order to pay for Obamacare can only be deleterious for the already frail Medicare environment. The

PPACA reduces the Medicare advantage program by $132 billion and decreases Medicare home health payments by forty billion and reduces Medicare hospital payments by thirteen billion.

I have already read the headlines regarding the decision of major corporations choosing to make all employees part-time workers in order to avoid payment for health insurance requirements for full-time employees under Obamacare. Several physicians have already told me of plans to opt out of Medicare in order to avoid possible audits and penalties administered under the auspices of Obamacare. It is also interesting that there are already reports of increased costs and excessive billing code utilizations, which have occurred under the required electronic medical record (EMR) stipulations of the PPACA. It turns out that it is easier for clerks to click the mouse for increasing the level of a consult in the EMR system than it was in the past when handwritten paperwork volume was needed to document levels of complexity.

There are wide variations as to the cost projections and effects relative to the budget deficit. Hopefully, these estimates are more accurate than the initial false projections concerning Medicare in 1965. A commonly raised concern about the cost projections of the PPACA is that the CBO (Congressional Budget Office) did not include the "doc fix" component into the cost projections, which will increase physician payments by over two hundred billion from 2012 to 2019. In 2010, the CBO stated, "Rising health costs will put tremendous pressure on the federal budget during the next few decades and beyond. In the CBO's judgment, the health legislation enacted earlier this year does not substantially diminish that pressure." In 2012, the CBO projected that the PPACA would require more than $1.7 trillion in gross federal spending for the decade of 2012–2022.

To summarize, it seems highly unlikely that the PPACA will result in cost savings and a reduced budget deficit with regard to national health-care spending. It is much more likely that the CBO has again underestimated the actual future costs of the program, given their dismal prior track record. In my opinion, top down regulatory attempts at cost controls, which is what Obamacare attempts to do, are additional producers of frustration for health-care providers but will likely be ineffective at decreasing costs or increasing access to medical professionals. In contrast, given the number of physicians threatening to retire or opt out of Medicare because of this law, I am very concerned that access to health-care professionals will likely become more constrained as the law becomes completely instituted.

MEDICAL MALPRACTICE CHALLENGES

One of my mentors aptly stated that neurosurgeons experience the highest of the highs and the lowest of the lows. As wonderful as it feels to cure someone from a previously incurable condition, there remains great frustration and emotional pain when you have to look a young man in the eyes and tell him his spinal cord is irreversibly damaged, and he will never walk again. Recently, I had to inform a mother of a two-year-old that the tumor I just removed successfully from her child was highly malignant and would require intense chemotherapy and likely damaging radiation therapy to have the best chance of preventing the tumor from recurring. It broke my heart to watch her fall limp to the floor in front of me, wailing in grief from the weight of the words I had just spoken to her. I had to remain calm and appear strong on the outside and give also the honest but tempered and hopeful words that we have achieved more long-term survivors lately and that he is in a relatively good prognostic group compared to some other children, but also clearly explain that there are no guarantees and unfortunately a significant risk of recurrence exists.

I have children of my own and inside my heart aches as I think of what my wife would be going through if this message had been given to us. The pain sinks in with the realization that from this moment onward, life is forever changed for this boy and his family. I and other doctors can often cope and deal with these situations, as difficult as they may be, because we recognize that we did not place that tumor in the child, and that it is not our fault. We are the good guys, trying to beat the evil monster. But for me personally, the worst and lowest of the lows occur when, while trying my best, something still went wrong and a complication occurred. Remorse, anguish, second-guessing, replaying the procedure over and over in my mind, and lost sleep are all common occurrences after such events. A young mother who had a stroke, resulting in hemiparesis, due to unknowingly sacrificing a tiny but critical artery during removal of a benign vascular malformation continues to haunt me to this day. Fortunately, these situations do not occur often, but unfortunately, there are others like her. Neurosurgeons I know have commented that the good outcomes erase from memory too quickly, but the bad ones linger in the mind seemingly forever. This may be partly because the cured patients these days, after minimally invasive approaches, often go home the next day; however, those with complications remain in the hospital and linger for days or weeks. They often develop secondary complications due to immobility, which further torments the physician's soul. Rounding to these patient's rooms each day is so tortuous emotionally that I would avoid it if I could, but the patient needs you more than ever when their condition has worsened, rather than improved, and there are inevitably many more painful questions by family members in these rooms to answer, so one has to stick it out and hang in there for the duration of the hospital stay and sometimes for years in the outpatient clinic. We have monthly morbidity and mortality conferences where every case is discussed among our peers to allow us to examine the cause of death or complication so that we may learn and especially teach the upcoming generation of physicians to avoid the same mistakes or consequences in the future.

I need to regress here for a moment and explain this process a bit more fully. I work in one of the busiest neurosurgical centers in the world where between six thousand and seven thousand neurosurgical procedures are performed each year. We discuss approximately thirty cases each month of people who have either died while on the neurosurgical service or suffered a complication as a result of a procedure. Simple math would conclude that $12 \times 30 = 660$ or about 10 percent of the cases each month are discussed. That sounds great compared to the days of Harvey Cushing, however is quite humbling for us to realize today. A bit of clarification is necessary. Most of the deaths discussed are patients who arrived at the hospital in a hopeless condition. As a junior resident, I remember feeling that I had chosen the most morbid profession in the world. I routinely performed brain death determinations almost every time I was on call for what seemed like an endless stream of poor souls who had suffered massive hemorrhages into their brains from ruptured aneurysms, motor vehicle accidents, gunshot wounds, uncontrolled hypertension, falls while taking anticoagulants, etc. So please understand that the majority of these morbidity and mortality cases, which are presented, are not the result of errors in medical judgment or bad technique.

Many complications are secondary to what I would call the natural consequences of life and underscore the relative frailty of the human body and challenging conditions that continue to frustrate our best attempts at interventions to date. By definition, someone who needs a neurosurgical operation of any kind is sick in one way or another. And sick patients come to us with various medical problems, which may or may not be related to, or a consequence of, the problem for which we are seeing them.

When I am talking to patients in clinic about their conditions and the possible surgical procedures recommended to them, I am required by law to discus with them the risks and possible complications they may encounter as a result of the procedure to be performed. I am also supposed to discuss the alternatives to the recommended procedure and explain rationally to them why I am recommending a certain procedure over another. We commonly discuss the "natural history" of their condition, meaning what is likely to happen if no intervention is undertaken. We must be able to support our recommendation with rational thought and sound medical data based on clinical research and published results of outcomes in similar people who have undergone the same recommended treatment. It must be understood that no two patients are exactly alike and the inherent risk of one patient, undergoing the same procedure, is not the same as another. It goes without saying that an otherwise healthy twenty-five-year-old has a very different risk of surgery compared to an eighty-year-old with diabetes and a history of previous cardiac infarction and renal insufficiency.

It also must be understood that no two conditions are exactly alike. Especially when it comes to the treatment of brain tumors, it is truly remarkable how different they are and how vastly different the risk of removal of one tumor is compared to another. Some tumors are truly benign and their removal is straightforward with a high probability of cure and a low risk of complication. But again, depending on the patient's health and general condition, even the simplest tumor removal can never be guaranteed to be resected without some risk of a complication or even death. Other tumors are in such difficult locations and involve vitally important functional areas of the brain, rendering any attempt at a complete removal in danger of leaving the patient with severe neurological deficits. Therefore, only a biopsy or limited resection of these tumors is recommended followed by some other adjunctive therapy, commonly some form of radiation or chemotherapy or both. Attempts at improving the outcomes for these patients are the subjects of countless publications in numerous medical journals. Much time is devoted at medical meetings and millions of dollars of research grants are awarded each year to improve the plight of patients with these malignant and invasive tumors. Unfortunately, some of the most common cancers to affect children arise in the brain, and most are, as of yet, incurable. We have made great strides at earlier detection with high resolution imaging techniques, namely MRI scanning, and the prognosis for some tumors has clearly improved over the years.

In the early days of Harvey Cushing, the mortality rate for brain tumors started out at about 50 percent. Before he developed his techniques of monitored anesthesia and sterile technique, nearly every patient died as a result of infection in the brain. As a result of his meticulous techniques and record keeping, the mortality rate by the end of his career approached 10 percent. Today, the operative mortality rate of an electively scheduled brain tumor operation is less than 1 percent. We take for granted now that everyone should make it through the operation in part due to the skill and expertise of our anesthesia colleagues. In fact to this day, after performing over 10,000 surgeries, and even in an extremely busy center like ours, intra-operative death is an amazingly rare event, which may only occur once a year or less. That is why I was so disappointed in an otherwise excellent movie *The Bucket List*. At the end of the movie, the character played by Morgan Freeman went into surgery for the removal of a brain metastasis, which is actually usually quite simple and straightforward, especially since he was completely coherent and appeared normal before the operation. However, he was portrayed to have died in the operating room. This is another example of media misrepresentation of reality. I suppose it made for good drama, but this just doesn't happen in the real word today. I have had to alleviate the fears of several patients and families to counteract the unnecessary fears caused by this misleading movie scene.

My children can tell you that they cannot watch medical shows on TV with me because there are generally so many misrepresentations and inconsistencies to be pointed out that it becomes unbearable. The general representation of medicine in the media, especially from news shows, which are often a form of free advertisement for some medical procedure, has the opposite effect of *The Bucket List*. It is portrayed that medical miracles exist for every ailment today and that all treatments are simple and painless and that stem cells and other innovations will all result in immortality for all of us in the near future. Any complication is depicted as secondary to negligence and could have and should have been completely avoided, if only the physicians would have been smarter, more caring, or more diligent. Worst of all today are the open advertisements of lawyers promising financial compensation for medical malpractice from physicians, pharmaceutical companies, or medical device manufacturers.

You can see where I am going with this. One primary problem with escalating health-care costs in America is the issue of medical malpractice. I have yet to speak to a single physician, conservative or liberal, primary care physician or specialist, who does not agree with me that lawsuit abuse is the most important problem to correct in order to curtail the cost of health care in America. There is a common joke enjoyed among physicians, which might be funnier if it did not feel so true to us. It goes something like this: "In France, you may die from chasing too many women. In Germany, you may die from drinking too much beer. In Spain, one might die being chased by bulls. But in America, if you die, it must be a doctor's fault!"

A recent case bears this point out. A cop, who was reportedly noncompliant with medications and life-style/diet recommendations from his cardiologist regarding blood pressure control, was scheduled for a cardiac stress test the following week but died of a heart attack while engaged in a sexual threesome, which did not include his wife. A jury awarded his wife a five-million-dollar malpractice award because the cardiologist allegedly did not warn the patient that sexual activity was risky in light of his coronary artery disease. As a token ruling, the award was decreased to three million dollars due to partial responsibility of the patient. This is ludicrous! The patient is and should be 100 percent responsible for his life decisions. His cardiologist didn't smoke, wasn't overweight, didn't have high blood pressure, and wasn't unfaithful to his wife. A jury may feel bad for the wife of this sexually adventurous police officer, but she married the guy and has some responsibility for that choice. The lottery winning award is costly to not only his cardiologist but to every one of us because it causes increased health-care costs. Small businesses cannot afford to provide health-care insurance for their employees because the premiums include compensation for ridiculous awards like this one. This death was not due to negligence or malpractice by his cardiologist, whether or not he mentioned anything about risks of sexual behavior. Where is the principal of personal responsibility and common sense?

There is no other country in the world that even closely approaches the extent of medical malpractice suits seen in America. When I attend international meetings, the foreign physicians seem almost oblivious to the concept of being sued and often ask questions regarding how different it must be to practice medicine in such a threatening environment. A 2001 study comparing the rates of malpractice claims between countries documented that the number of claims were 350 percent higher in America compared to Canada.

There has been much written about the potential cost containment, which may result from tort reform. As in all things, it is very important to examine the source of the information regarding anything written on this issue. During the political debates of the 2008 election, whenever this topic came up, wide variations in cost-saving projections were quoted. You don't have to be a cynic to recognize the political influence of money in the form of campaign contributions and their relationship to information on this subject. The Association of Trail Lawyers of America (ATLA) was recently renamed the American Association for Justice (AAJ) presumably to disconnect this group from an obviously poor general reputation and connotation of the label "Trial Lawyers." The ATLA-AAJ has consistently been a heavy hitter in the ring of political lobbying. They have contributed a total of over thirty-six million dollars to both political parties since financial records were made public in 1990; however, the AAJ was reportedly the number one single contributor to the Democratic Party with donations totaling nearly thirty-two million dollars since 1990. Interestingly, during the 2012 election cycle, when the Republicans voiced interest in supporting Tort reform, the AAJ did not given any money to what they felt was a lost cause in the republican party, but continued to pour money into the Democratic party, presumably because they still believed that they had significant influence among the Democratic lawmakers. The AAJ boasts an international membership of fifty-six thousand members, but this also includes paralegals and law students. This group of highly paid and influential lawyers has been holding the entire country hostage with regard to the malpractice issue. It is most likely that because of the extent of their political contributions, every time the issue of tort reform came up, it was simply discarded and claimed to be off the table for discussion or, at best, given lip service and then promised to be discussed more thoroughly at a later date. Studies were quoted that stated that only a very small amount of money would be saved since only 0.5 percent of health-care dollars are actually spent on malpractice insurance. This estimate grossly underestimates the true costs of the malpractice climate in the United States.

I will cite one well-known example of a prominent trial lawyer who made so much money by litigating physicians that he was able to make a bid for the presidency. John Edwards made his fortune from lawsuits against obstetricians for alleging and successfully convincing the courts that these physicians were guilty of negligence in their handling of complicated deliveries. Such alleged negligence supposedly resulted in the development of cerebral palsy in these children. Mr. Edwards's payment for this bit of legal expertise was over sixty-five million dollars. This case has been analyzed and scrutinized extensively. The millions of dollars paid out to Mr. Edwards were mere drops in the bucket compared to the resultant increased medical costs for obstetrics in America. The malpractice insurance required to cover physicians for obstetrical care skyrocketed. Family physicians could no longer afford malpractice insurance to cover their occasional delivery of babies of their established patients. This especially affected the care and handling of pregnancies in rural areas. Access to obstetrics in many states became severely limited, and in many counties, there were no physicians offering obstetrical care, period! Women were forced to cross state lines and seek care in major medical centers at significant distances away from their homes. This obviously resulted in higher overall risks for the entire population because of the lack of local access and lack of personalized care. The risk for true emergency deliveries became higher because of the time needed for travel to a hospital offering obstetrical services. The percentage of cesarean sections compared to routine deliveries increased dramatically after these litigations. In some centers the rate of C-sections increased fivefold within just a few years of this legal decision. Interestingly, the rate of cerebral palsy did not change one iota as a result of the increased number of cesarean sections. It has since been shown that millions of women have undergone unnecessary C-sections as a direct result of the legal climate and hysteria created by this infamous trial lawyer. Even to this day, advertisements soliciting suits for supposed negligence in cases of cerebral palsy with the promise of generous compensation are seen in all forms of media.

If you listen to or watch the videos sponsored by the AAJ, they will portray themselves as the only voice sticking up for the little guy against the wealthy corporations and insurance companies. They are the ones preserving your rights to sue your physician if he or she injures you by means of malpractice. They are the advocates for the poor, the needy, and the underrepresented insuring your right to trial by jury. Is there some truth to their claims and can you be persuaded by their position? Of course, it sounds good and is admirable in principle. Unfortunately, the greed principle has overtaken most of the admirable notions in practice. The pendulum has swung so far to the side of being able to sue for injustice that there is no longer any sense of personal responsibility but rather potential lottery winnings for any unfortunate outcome, no matter the underlying cause. Several Seinfeld episodes come to mind in which Kramer solicits the help of the civil litigator Jackie Chiles for help in various frivolous lawsuits. It made for great comedy, but as in many things, art imitates real life, and it is only funny because it reflects in part the true nature of the situation at hand.

Please understand that I am in no way suggesting that there should be no means to police or punish gross negligence on the part of physicians or any developer or manufacturer of drugs or devices. Indeed, *if* there is clear and convincing evidence that a company purposefully ignored verifiable data, which suggested a substantial risk in a large population of patients who may receive a drug, then that company should receive substantial punishment. Innocently harmed patients as a result of their negligence should be entitled to some degree of compensation. After writing these sentences, I feel much more like a lawyer than a doctor and that makes me very uncomfortable. I did, however, choose my words somewhat carefully. First and foremost, *if* is a very big word. What constitutes clear and convincing evidence and what is substantial punishment and what is appropriate compensation for someone's life or injury? These are all difficult questions, which are generally left up to the courts to decide. I wish to digress a little into some additional difficulties in this regard.

First of all, there is the issue of complexity. The more that I have studied the human brain, and even more so the molecular basis of life and diseases, I am simply astounded at the complexity of it all. Anyone who has attempted to memorize the Krebs cycle, involved with cellular energy and metabolism and the numerous enzymes activated and deactivated along the way for a cell to utilize consumed fuel for cellular functions, has gained some insight into what I am referring to. The replication and decoding of DNA, for cellular division and which serves as the blueprint for all of life's processes, is absolutely astounding in its complexity. Neuroscientists spend entire careers in the study of a single neurotransmitter receptor. The understanding of interactions and modulators of neurotransmitters and synapses due to these molecules, which serve a gateway for ions into and out of our brain cells, is unbelievably complex. They are ultimately responsible for electrical currents and transmission of information and yes, even thoughts, from our billions of brain cells.

Given this backdrop, isn't it astounding that we can ingest a chemical in the form of a pill and that those dissolved molecules become transported through the bloodstream and achieve a satisfactory concentration in the correct location along cellular membranes in the joints, the liver, or even the brain to have a measurable and even clinically detectable effect? The fact that we can even now design molecules to have specific and desired effects in this regard is astounding. However, it is absolutely inconceivable that an agent could be designed to have a specifically targeted effect without at least some degree of undesired or unknown effects. Now, so far, I have only alluded to the complexity within a single individual. Now think of the genetic variability within a population of people. There are many variable attributes, which we can see, such as physical stature, hair and eye color; but there are many more variations in our molecular basis that are not apparent to the eye but that may be apparent in their responses to medications. Side effects can be relatively standard and even predictable within "normal" people due to the known consequences of a certain medication of relatively specific intended targets but also widespread less specific unintended targets, which react to the same molecule in an undesired way. For example, the powerful steroidal anti-inflammatories like prednisone and dexamethasone predictably cause undesired weight gain and thinning of the skin in most people. However, there are substantial variations in the degree of this undesired response. Some people will gain over a hundred pounds and develop stretch marks while others gain only five to ten pounds over the same time period. Then there are the rare idiosyncratic reactions to medications, which only affect a small minority of patients and for whom there may be no warning that something may occur prior to exposure to the medication. The degree of relative risk only becomes known *after* enough people have been exposed and adversely affected. An example of this is malignant hyperthermia, which can be a fatal reaction to commonly used anesthetics, but which only affects about one in ten thousand people. It is such a rare occurrence that anesthesiologists and OR staffs may never see a case of it, but nevertheless, run drills and checks and put up laminated cheat sheets of what to do to maintain awareness of the possibility, in case they ever do.

So the question arises, "If one person is adversely affected by a medication, but 9,999 people benefit from that same medication, should that medication be banned from use? What if the ratio is 1:999, 1:99, 1:9, or 1:9,999,999?" Obviously, the answer depends on how bad the adverse reactions are and if there are other safer alternatives with equal efficacy. But what if there are no other options? What if the absence of the questioned medication or treatment results in suffering and even death of the 99 because of the fear of risk of treatment for the 1? These are real-life everyday issues facing the medical profession today. This is why the daytime-TV lawyer solicitation advertisements are so maddening. There is not a single treatment, procedure, medication, or device which can be guaranteed safe and effective for 100 percent of people. If class action law suits are based on rare idiosyncratic reactions for the few and result in the excessive expense and unavailability of treatments, devices, medications for the many, than we all suffer, and that is what is currently occurring. We are all paying exorbitantly for the lottery winnings of the few and are risking the suffering, not just monetarily, but literally suffering for the many.

One relatively recent example of this problem involves a class of anti-inflammatory medications known as COX-2 inhibitors. The common over-the-counter anti-inflammatory medication ibuprofen, with trade names Advil or Motrin, works by blocking the COX-1 and COX-2 enzymes involved in the inflammatory cascade of reactions. The medication is effective at decreasing pain and swelling by limiting this inflammatory response to a whole host of injuries and insults to the body. I have certainly taken advantage of this wonderful medical discovery after countless weekend warrior activities. Unfortunately, the COX-1 enzyme also is involved with normal process of providing the stomach lining with a protective coating. Therefore, blocking this enzyme also results in an increased risk of stomach ulcers by diminishing this protective coating. Some people are much more sensitive to this undesired effect than others and cannot take this medication for this reason.

Years ago, pharmaceutical researchers began the development of molecules, which would selectively block only the COX-2 enzyme and not the COX-1 enzyme in hopes of avoiding this side effect. The result was the development of medications with trade names including Vioxx and Celebrex. These medications were touted as being safer and more effective and were an excellent example of scientifically designed drugs aimed at a specific purpose. I had many patients take these medications for chronic back pain and postsurgical pain and found them to be effective especially for those whose stomach issues prevented them from using the cheaper ibuprofen. However, an unexpected side effect occurred with these medications. It was found after many years of use in millions of patients that there was a higher risk of myocardial infarction (heart attack) among those patients who used these drugs regularly for long periods of time.

Prostaglandins are molecules involved in the inflammatory cascade, which are blocked by these drugs and is the mechanism for decreasing pain and swelling. However, some good prostaglandins are also blocked, more selectively, by the more precise COX-2 inhibitors, and this allegedly results in lipid build up in the arteries and an increased risk of atherosclerosis (hardening and narrowing of the arteries) which leads to heart attacks and strokes. Vioxx was particularly implicated in this and in one report was suggested to have lead to over twenty-seven thousand heart attacks or sudden cardiac deaths. Due to these studies, the drug was pulled from the market and class action lawsuits were filed. There was an implication that the drug company Merck had suppressed or ignored some evidence of increased cardiac risk in the initial trials of the drug. It is uncertain if the cardiac risk is specific to Vioxx or is related to all drugs of this class. Celebrex remains on the market but carries a warning of possible increased cardiac risk. Celebrex was reported to have been used by over seventy-five million people as of 2001 without any evidence of increased cardiac events. The studies to elucidate causality after millions of people have been using a drug in the general public are very difficult to interpret.

These medications are used primarily in patients with arthritis and of course patients with arthritis are generally elderly. Heart attacks are very common in this age group, comprising the second most common cause of death. Therefore, determining a significant additional causality of an arthritis medication retrospectively can be quite difficult. What if arthritis by itself is associated with an increased risk of cardiac disease, with or without these medications? Arthritis is an inflammatory disease. The build up of plaques in arteries also involves inflammation, so it is not unreasonable to assume that patients who take these drugs may already have an increased risk of a cardiac event.

Interestingly, aspirin blocks some of the same prostaglandins in the inflammatory cascade and has a significant antiplatelet effect. The platelets are the small fragmented constituents in blood, which seal leaks and stop bleeding by forming clumps over small holes from inside the blood vessels. They are activated by inflammation and are particularly sensitive to raw surfaces or plaques in vessels. It is actually a platelet plug formed on the inner vessel surface plaque of a narrowed vessel, which results in the blockage of the vessel and causes the heart attack. Aspirin, by blocking this platelet aggregation, significantly reduces this risk of heart attacks and strokes. It also explains why people who take aspirin regularly are more prone to bruising and bleeding. Sometimes, serious internal bleeding, including fatal brain hemorrhages occur because people are taking aspirin. It has been suggested that if aspirin were a new drug, it would never gain FDA clearance because of the multiple side effects and drug interactions associated with it.

Ibuprofen and other nonsteroidal ant-inflammatory drugs also have antiplatelet effects, but to a much smaller degree compared to aspirin. It therefore comes as bit of a surprise that the selective COX-2 inhibitors would have been implicated in increasing rather than decreasing platelet aggregation and increasing rather than decreasing risks of heart attacks.

The above example of the COX-2 inhibitor saga gives us much to discuss regarding the role of legal threats and development of new medically useful agents and devices, and we will return to this later.

Secondly, beyond the issue of complexity is a fundamental problem in human nature and our thought processes regarding a tendency to draw conclusions prematurely and with minimal evidence. Numerous recent studies and books have been published regarding the above statement. I encourage the reader to further explore these well-written articles and books on this subject. In brief, we humans developed a rapid, but often inaccurate, decision-making process through evolutionary history. The premise can be summed up in the presumed observation that: "because he who ran from the bear first survived, whereas, he who sat and logically contemplated his options more slowly and logically was eaten and thus did not pass along that tendency in his genes." This is of course an oversimplification. However, it is a useful starting point of the discussion. Rapid, emotionally based decisions were favored in a survival of the fittest environment whereas our environment has changed radically over the past few centuries into an extremely complex and more crowded, socially networking world.

Humans are generally quite curious and have an innate need for explanations to observed phenomena. Just think of your favorite three-year-old after he or she has discovered the word *why*. However, most of us, and certainly individuals of the past, seem to have been relatively easily satisfied with any explanation to the question at hand, which seemed the least bit plausible. The ancient Greeks, known for tremendous advances in the understanding of mathematics, medicine, architecture, democracy, etc., were satisfied with many of the harder questions of life by attributing them to the whims of their humanized mythical gods. Many of them truly believed that the stars in the heavens were holes in the overlying fabric above of the earth, separating them from the world of the gods.

We want to know answers to questions, but it appears that we are quick to fixate on any easily obtained semi-plausible answer and hold to that belief, seeking any evidence to confirm it, but denying, or ignoring evidence to the contrary, once an opinion or decision has been made. The sci-fi classic Star Trek explored this idea rather well comparing the purely logically thinking Spock to the emotionally reacting but highly effective Captain Kirk. I am chagrinned to have seen my childhood hero Kirk (William Shattner) as a spokesman for a malpractice law firm's TV advertisement. I'll get back to the point. It takes work, patience, time and effort, and brainpower to think logically and rationally. It is generally faster, more efficient, and even often right to follow hunches and respond to the first choice our brain comes up with. But often right, doesn't mean always right.

Neurosurgeons are typically surmised as being "sometimes wrong, but never in doubt." People want quick and easy answers and explanations, not long and drawn-out theories. I am asked at least once a week, "What causes brain tumors?" The key word to contemplate here is *cause*. I typically frame my response to this question relative to the degree of education and background of the person asking the question. Truth be known, there really isn't any known direct cause. It involves a complex cellular/biochemical mistake in the chromosomal replication of glial progenitor cells. But what caused that? We often erroneously state that smoking *causes* lung cancer. It would be much more correct to say that smoking is associated with a much higher incidence of lung cancer in people who smoke, compared to the nonsmoking population. As much as I hate smoking and as emotional as it is to treat a young person in his late twenties with multiple metastatic brain tumors who started smoking when he was nine, my temptation and usual phraseology is to use the *cause* word. However, strictly speaking, there was some genetic difference within this unfortunate young man, which allowed him to be much more susceptible to the carcinogenic chemicals in cigarettes compared to George Burns who proudly still smoked on his one hundredth birthday without lung cancer. It also is important for us to remind ourselves that a small percentage of lung cancer victims never smoked. So what caused it in them? Evil secondhand smoke is implicated in some, no doubt, but what about others?

Some of my patients are convinced that cell phones caused their brain tumor because it was on the same side of their brain that they used their cell phone. But remember, it is a fifty-fifty chance. There have been numerous studies, some of which I have been well informed of, which have convincing evidence that there is no increased association of cell phone use with brain tumors. It is comforting to know that electromagnetic wave frequencies used in cell phone technology, similar to microwaves and radio waves, typically do not have sufficient energy to make DNA strand breaks, like ionizing radiation does. Genetic mutations caused by breakage of DNA strands and erroneous repair of these breaks are the best understood underlying mechanisms and cause of carcinogenesis. The proximity to the ears would also mean that there should be a much higher risk of skin cancers to the ear itself, which we do not see, as compared to brain tumors. But again, regardless, of evidence or logic, people can remain convinced of a cause and effect.

We want things to be black or white, right or wrong. We don't do well with shades of gray. It takes too much time to really understand an issue, so we become naturally complacent and satisfied with sound bites and gravitational polarizing statements, which agree with our first hunches and are much less likely to really put forth the effort to find out the truth of a matter. We tend to see things from our own biased perspective. Have you ever listened to avid fans in any sporting event? The fans reactions to the referee's calls are so inherently biased that it becomes comical if you are an unbiased observer. There have actually been detailed neuropsychiatrical studies showing that the way our brains reconstruct an event, like at a ball game, makes us literally see the event with a bias favorable to our emotional attachment relative to the event. Think of that the next time your tennis opponent calls your ace serve out. He may not actually be consciously cheating, only subconsciously cheating. Mothers have a very hard time accepting even the most obvious evidence, which might implicate the guilt of their child in a crime. Our own brains employ an amazing assortment of defense mechanisms to defend our acceptance of fault or responsibility with regard to an unwanted event or action.

I have attempted to introduce this fallacy of human nature in order to apply it to the problem at hand. Medicine operates in the shades of gray. It is filled with statistics and probabilities and even a high degree of randomness and occasional improbabilities. I am often struck by the surprise case of something I have never seen before, in spite of now many years of experience. It makes life, and my job, challenging and interesting. It is truly never the same. Sure, some cases become relatively routine, or even mundane, in their repetition. However, every case must be evaluated in the context of occurring within a unique individual.

There is a great push to standardize treatments and diagnosis and attempt to take out the human variability and biases among physicians. There is currently a major push in the medical community to subject as many of our treatment decisions as possible to a standard of level 1 scientific evidence. Level 1 scientific evidence means that a treatment has been tested in a clinical trial in a double-blinded, randomized, placebo-controlled fashion. However, as much as we try to do this as a medical profession, and as admirable as our goals may be, not all treatment decisions can be subjected to this kind of testing. Many standard therapies have become so ingrained and presumed true that it would be considered unethical to subject them to a randomized controlled trial because half of the patients would be purposely denied standard care in such a trial. The most common analogy for this point is to sarcastically suggest that there should be a randomized controlled trial to prove the efficacy of parachutes for skydivers. Who would want to jump out of the plane in a study with a 50 percent chance of not having a parachute?

Medicine and life, and all of nature for that matter, is subject to randomness and improbabilities. I therefore conclude and propose that it is impossible to predict all outcomes to medical intervention. It is ludicrous to expect 100 percent safety and 0 percent risk for any medical intervention. Standard of care is a continuously fluid entity and will always depend on some degree of human error and interpretation.

In my field of neurosurgery, the risk of missing a diagnosis is considered so high that any thought of avoiding a test is usually discounted because the amount of money saved in not ordering a test is negligible compared to the potential dollars at risk from a malpractice claim, which may result from not ordering a test, even if the possibility of a positive test is only a fraction of a percent. Emergency room physicians feel especially vulnerable in this regard. I am certain that not a day goes by in any major city emergency room without a kid being brought in because of a fall or sport injury with a bump on the head, possibly accompanied by symptoms of a mild concussion. Nearly every one of these children undergoes a CT scan of the head at a cost of about $1,000 and with a resultant exposure to radiation. The overwhelming majority of these CT scans are negative, and even if they are technically positive in showing a trace amount of blood, or a nondisplaced skull fracture, nothing other than simple observation and comfort measures are required for their treatment. In other words, probably 999 out of a thousand of these scans can be considered technically unnecessary and offered no real value to the patient but resulted in significant medical costs to be born by the family or their insurance company.

However, for the picture as a whole, one thousand normal CT scans to find one life-threatening scan is actually a valid investment. Let me rationalize in malpractice terms. There is a well-known possible serious result of head trauma, which occurs especially in the young called an epidural hematoma. An expanding epidural hematoma in a young person is a true neurosurgical emergency. A teenager can literally be awake and talking to you in one minute and then an hour later be in a deep coma and suffer irreversible brain damage or death resulting from the expansion of this blood clot, which is typically induced by a skull fracture. The skull fracture may be relatively small but may cause a tear in an artery in the dura.

The dura is a protective membrane over the brain directly under the skull. In young people, this dural membrane can separate relatively easily from the overlying skull, to which it is usually adhered, due to the pressure of arterial blood pumping into this potential space. The expansion of this blood clot in the epidural space causes a displacement of the brain tissue and leads to what is called a herniation syndrome. The compressed brain herniates over toward the other side of the skull and in the process squeezes arteries and nerves resulting in decreased blood flow to the brain and damage to the compressed nerves. An ominous clinical finding of a seriously injured patient is a dilated and nonreactive pupil on one side, which means the third cranial nerve on that side of the brain has been compressed or otherwise injured. I have personally operated on many such cases, as have all trained neurosurgeons, and it is truly scary to know that less than an hour can make the difference between a normal life and a chronic vegetative survivor or dead patient.

There was a recent example of this tragic outcome in a celebrity, which made international news involving Natasha Richardson, who starred opposite Dennis Quaid, in one of my wife's favorite movie remakes, *The Parent Trap*. She suffered a head injury while skiing. She ultimately died of a herniation syndrome from an expanding epidural hematoma under her skull. I know nothing about the case except what was portrayed in the news; however, it seems that her death could have been avoided if she had been taken initially to a hospital with neurosurgical capabilities. The extra several hours required to transport her to a major medical center to receive surgery, after the diagnosis was made at a smaller hospital, resulted in irreversible brain injury before the clot could be removed to relieve the pressure off of her brain.

Now, let us go back to the rationalization for one thousand unnecessary tests. There have been successful malpractice suits for missing such epidural hematomas with awards typically being paid out, which are several millions of dollars, for alleged negligence in not promptly diagnosing and treating such patients.

Parenthetically, the surgical bill for performing such an operation is typically a few thousand dollars. Some surgeons have questioned why saving a life is only worth a few thousand dollars, but if one looses a life as a result of malpractice, that same life may be worth ten million dollars. So if a thousand CT scans cost a thousand dollars each, the sum of all these scans equals approximately one million dollars. Therefore, it is actually cost effective to order excessive CT scans from a defensive medicine point of view. However, it becomes even more complicated than this.

I am aware of a case where a CT scan was obtained which did show a small epidural hematoma in an otherwise completely normal boy. It was elected to not perform the surgery to repair the fracture and coagulate the torn artery because on several repeated CT scans, the hematoma did not expand and the patient had no symptoms. After several days of observation and multiple repeated scans without any change in the size of the hematoma, the young man was sent home and instructed to follow up with yet another scan in a week. Tragically, he may have had another minor fall or event at home, which may have caused the bleeding to restart on a delayed basis, and he died as a result. As expected, the family under the admonition of a trial lawyer sought for millions in reparations for this "malpractice."

I find it most ironic that the surgeon actually gets paid for operations performed and receives no compensation for choosing not to operate and takes all the risks by not doing so. This surgeon who was sued (unsuccessfully in this case) has informed me that he has serious doubts as to whether he will ever simply observe and not prophylactically operate on a similar case in the future. I personally have managed many such cases with small skull fractures and small epidural hematomas nonoperatively, which never resulted in a bad outcome, and I have felt good about not subjecting a child to an unnecessary operation. However, I may have been sued for making the exact same decision if the outcome had been different.

There is truth to the adage, "Damned if you do, damned if you don't." If a surgeon makes it his policy to operate on every patient with such a condition defensively to avoid even the slightest risk of a bad outcome as a result of not operating, he will sooner or later have a patient suffer a significant complication as a result of a surgery he performed. He may even indeed be sued for performing an unnecessary surgery. Even with today's excellent anesthesia techniques, there are occasional unexpected complications, which may occur even in otherwise healthy individuals. The anesthesiologist may drop a lung (pneumothorax) as a result of placing a central line, which is placed due to the possibility of significant blood loss in order to give rapid fluid resuscitation. That same central line may cause line sepsis or thrombophlebitis. Urinary tract infections secondary to Foley catheter insertions, deep venous thrombosis, and malignant hyperthermia due to idiosyncratic reactions to the anesthetic agents are all added risks by taking a patient to surgery, which are avoided by the decision for observation. So that is the crux of the question. What constitutes medical malpractice and what is an unfortunate bad outcome, which occurred due to "bad luck" in spite of acceptable and sound medical decision making?

There are other long-term issues, which need to be considered in this debate. By performing countless CT scans in order to find the one in a thousand positive finding, we are exposing patients to the long-term risks of ionizing radiation. Radiological biologists have reported a small but measurable increase in a lifetime cancer risk of a child who receives a single CT scan compared to children who were never scanned. It is not infeasible that in the future a class action lawsuit will be advertised on TV soliciting cancer victims with promises of significant financial compensation if they were administered a CT scan twenty years earlier. The lawyers will paint the ER physicians and hospital administrators as greedy and evil in their ordering and providing an unnecessary test with high risks, which resulted in their development of cancer. In plain terms, the lawyers want to be able to sue you if you don't order tests and sue you if you do. They want to sue you for not performing surgery and to sue you for surgery performed defensively. They are the ultimate Monday morning quarterbacks in a fantasy football league playing with our money, with nothing to lose, and everything to gain no matter which play is made.

I believe it is impossible to accurately estimate the excess costs added to the medical budget resulting from the practice of defensive medicine. There are simply no means to evaluate the underlying reasons for when a test is ordered or a when a surgical procedure is performed. As in the previously sited example of obstetrics, prior to the landslide changes resultant from the malpractice suit of John Edwards, fewer tests and fewer C-sections were performed. Because of a fear of physician litigation, and not due to sound medical judgment and practice, countless additional admissions for fetal heart monitoring and unnecessary C-sections were performed without any measurable decline in the rate of cerebral palsy. How does one accurately measure the increased costs in this and other similar situations?

The lawyers, of course, feel that they are providing a great service to patients in that they not only provide means for compensation for those who are injured but also provide a protection for future patients from injury by being a deterrent to negligent actions of all physicians, pharmaceutical companies, and biomedical manufacturers. There may obviously be some truth to this positional statement, however, much has been written about the tremendous inconsistencies and flaws inherent to our current tort system.

It has been shown that only a small fraction of patients are actually benefitted from the current system and that the judgments rendered are tremendously variable and don't follow any consistent pattern. This is especially true of the compensation for noneconomical expenses like placing a price tag on pain and suffering. The payouts for potential future earnings are also highly variable depending on the vocation and education of the injured patient. I have already addressed the issue of the threat of litigation being a deterrent to negligence. It certainly does act as a major deterrent, but it does so at such exorbitant costs and with such far-reaching additional effects as alluded to above that it is probably ultimately causing much more harm than good in the number of excessive tests and procedures, which are performed to defend against the possibility of being sued.

Therefore, lawsuits and the resultant monetary payouts need to be limited exclusively to cases of true medical fraud and gross negligence. There must be a broad-based societal understanding and agreement that by limiting lawsuit abuse, the availability of medical treatment will be increased for the masses. The number of unnecessary tests and procedures will decrease along with the complications and costs associated with these tests. The overall cost of medicine will decrease for the many *if* this change in philosophy is adopted and sustained over time. However, because an entire generation of physicians has been trained in the current litigious environment, it may take a significant amount of time for the cost reductions to be realized.

I have observed that the residents who train in our institution have almost no conscious awareness of the defensive medicine they are practicing or of the high costs of the tests and procedures they are ordering. The real problem is that there are almost no incentives against ordering a test, and the ordering physician protects himself from liability by doing so. The physician, by not ordering a test, may be saving someone else's money but at a perceived potentially career-ending cost to him. This is really the crux of the problem. Currently, there is a complete disconnect between the person at risk for the possibility of malpractice and the person paying the bills to prevent the potential risk. Market pressures can never correct this problem within the current framework of medical economics.

It has been suggested that a better and more equitable system would be to set up a "complication fund" for the benefit of all unfortunate patients with unexpectedly bad outcomes after medical procedures, not necessarily tied to fault or issues of malpractice. A small (say a 1–2 percent tax on all invasive procedures) could be set aside for these individuals. The compensation would be modest and limited to provide for care needed as a result of the complication and for modest living expenses or long-term care assistance if necessary. Those who would qualify for such funds would be evaluated by an appointed board of medical experts and social workers. If such a program were instituted, a more compassionate and broad-based effort to assist those with complications could occur rather than a haphazard lottery winning for a few.

There is a secondary problem that has occurred because of medical liability risks from those who have no insurance. Large hospitals in urban centers are particularly vulnerable and are in severe trouble today because of the high proportion of patients presenting to the emergency rooms who have no insurance. Trauma centers have a government stipulation for requirement of coverage from all the major subspecialties such as orthopedic surgery, neurosurgery, general surgery, anesthesiology, cardiology, etc. This requirement for specialty coverage is necessary to ensure that all serious life-threatening conditions can be adequately treated if patients requiring these services are flown in by helicopter on any given day and at any given time during the day. This requires specialists to be on call at the hospital and available within a short amount of time.

Traditionally, surgical specialists are required to take call at that hospital in order to have privileges to admit patients and to perform surgery at that hospital. It is well-known that within the current system, surgical charges from the operating rooms and cardiology suites are the largest moneymakers for the hospital. The high amount of revenue generated from these procedures has subsidized many other departments of hospitals for years and has provided the ability to offer care for the indigent.

Currently, however, when up to 40 percent of patients who present to the emergency room have no insurance and no means to pay for services rendered and have the ability to sue physicians who may treat them, physicians are taking a significant financial risk by being on call and assuming the care for these patients. When a specialist is on call for the emergency room, he has agreed to accept the responsibility of care for all patients who come in during his period of call. In the past, when most patients had insurance, this was a good thing, and young enthusiastic specialists, fresh out of residency training, would gladly take call in order to build up practice and generate income. This was a win-win situation for the hospital as well. However with the aspect of uninsured patients and because of the EMTALA law, it is realized that the physicians are taking more of a financial risk than they are potentially going to earn by taking hospital call. Because of this financial predicament, currently hospitals have to subsidize specialists and pay them a stipend of typically one thousand to three thousand dollars daily simply to take call at these hospitals.

In the past, there were no other options for surgeons other than large full-service hospitals to operate in. However, now, large groups of physicians have invested in surgical centers, which are completely equipped with the latest hospital equipment and provide excellent care and facilities for insured patients. These surgical centers do not have any emergency rooms and only accept patients for surgery within their facilities after they have been preapproved by their insurance company with a guaranteed payment for services rendered. Physicians who have invested in the development and operation of these surgical centers have found this situation to be highly lucrative because they can receive income from their surgical fees as well as from the surgical center's charges for the facility use. Patients who are treated in these centers are typically very pleased with the high level of service they receive and the centers typically get very high marks on patient satisfaction surveys. Many surgeons who operate in these centers no longer bother to take call in traditional hospitals because they can shield themselves from a significant amount of liability as well as from the late-night drama of drunken and disorderly patients who would not have paid them anyway.

The development of these surgical centers may have been a great boon to surgical specialists; however, this has had a terrible impact on traditional urban hospitals. Not only have the centers sucked away some of the best specialists, they have also taken all of the dollars that they generated with their privately insured patients with them. The result is truly disastrous because even a higher percentage of uninsured patients and undocumented immigrants are being treated in these urban hospitals compared to the past when there was a significant influx of insured patients. At one point, our large group of over twenty neurosurgeons considered building and managing our own specialty hospital because of the financial advantages described above. However, we realized that the hospital in which we work, which is the oldest and largest in Arizona, would never survive without us. In good conscience, we decided to stay within the traditional hospital system and try to make things work. However, it remains an extreme challenge; and our hospital is currently running in the red, losing millions of dollars per quarter.

FLAWED COST-SAVING ATTEMPTS

Health insurance companies are currently applying significant pressure on physicians to limit the number of tests and procedures performed on their patients. Every clinically active physician is feeling this pressure in the form of increasingly numerous hoops and hurdles and forms and phone calls needed for authorization prior to any significant test or surgical procedure. The insurance companies employ physicians as medical directors whose primary occupation is to review proposed tests and procedures and deny their authorization unless the ordering physician can support the need based on accepted medical literature. This process is time consuming, costly, frustrating, and extremely annoying from the treating physician's perspective. Indeed, surgeons typically employ one or two office staff personnel with their primary job description being to obtain these medical authorizations. The more aggressive medical directors don't simply listen to the doctor's staff but demand a personal phone call from the surgeon to plead his case for the patient who needs the procedure. Having participated in this process numerous times, I have found this process to be an absolutely maddening waste of time and energy. The reader should be made aware that these physicians who have taken employment from the insurance companies in this capacity are typically former general practitioners who view their jobs as an easier alternative, almost a type of retirement, compared to the clinical practice of medicine. They are armed with medical literature search engines on the Internet but with very limited personal knowledge or experience about the proposed procedure or the indications to perform it. In fact, most internists, family practitioners, and emergency room physicians have never spent a single day on a neurosurgical service in their entire medical training. Therefore, they are in no position to decide who is or is not in need of a procedure or test. They have not seen the patient and may have no clue what the actual medical condition is, or the indications for tests or procedures to try to diagnose or treat it. The medical director gains employment by the insurance company for one purpose, and that is to slow or obstruct the outflow of money from their employer by making it more difficult for procedures to be performed. The insurance company is actually making medical decisions without seeing the patients, and they are attempting to deny tests and procedures, which are ordered by board certified doctors, who have seen and examined the patients. It is obvious that this strategy is functioning, at least in part, because these medical directors may actually make more money in this capacity as obstructionists than they do caring for patients themselves. How sad and ironic is that?

Because I am considered a financial "softie" in the group, I have been figuratively called to the "principal's office" for semisecretively accepting patients, which were not on our accepted insurance plans for very specialized care, which is really not available elsewhere. I have learned however that by so doing, I was actually enabling the insurance executives to continue to not provide adequate coverage for their clients needs. It should be a crime for an insurance company CEO to pocket a personal bonus of twenty-five million dollars, which is obtained primarily from accepting insurance premiums from potentially needy patients but then effectively denying the needed care from qualified physicians and pocketing the unspent money. I personally find it absolutely absurd that a CEO of United Healthcare was reported to have personally pocketed 101 million dollars in stock options due to financial manipulations of the insurance company. It is certainly a conflict of interest to have stock holders and insurance company bottom lines held to a higher standard than the delivery of compassionate care to health-care consumers of insurance. What is the mission statement of an insurance company? Clearly in this case, it was to make the most money possible for those in positions of power and not to provide the best possible care for their client/patients.

The consumer of insurance, especially when the insurance is provided by the employer, is usually clueless, or at least profoundly unaware, about what extent of coverage they really have until the need arises for specialized medical treatment. Simply stated, the insurance company is required to provide all standard medical care including specialists such as neurosurgeons, should the need arise. However, they are not required to provide the best care available, only care from any fully credentialed specialist. Many people may be unaware about contracted rates of service between medical providers and insurance companies. Some insurance companies simply go with the lowest bidder. The lowest bidder is usually the provider who is not very busy and needs to undercut other more established specialists in order to grow his or her practice. Now this is a type of market force that could actually be seen as a positive, with respect to cost control. However, the person saving the money is the insurance executive and not the recipient of care. The person in need of the care never had a say in the matter since it was decided long before he or she ever knew that he would need this kind of care. The lowest bidder provider may indeed be very well qualified and an excellent physician, possibly recently moved into a new area or fresh out of residency. But he also may not be very busy because he is generally known to be substandard by his peers, who chose not to refer patients to that provider. I am certain that most individuals when they are choosing a physician for treatment would find it unsettling to discover that the specialist was only referred to because he was the lowest bidder on an insurance plan and not because the specialist was personally known to be a competent and caring physician who was knowledgeable, up-to-date, and especially qualified to treat the condition for which the care is needed.

As medicine has advanced, it has become impossible for one physician to be knowledgeable or skilled in every area of medicine. People generally understand that there needs to be specialists, but what most laypeople don't know is that even within specialties like neurosurgery there are many areas of subspecialization. For example, we have members in our group who subspecialize in spine, vascular, endovascular, skull base tumors, stereotactic radiosurgery, neurosurgical oncology, pain, movement disorders, pituitary tumors, pediatric neurosurgery, endoscopic neurosurgery, minimally invasive neurosurgery, epilepsy surgery, etc. It is absolutely impossible for one neurosurgeon to remain competent and up-to-date in all of these areas. Each of these subspecialty areas has associated journals and meetings and societies dedicated to furthering the knowledge and competence of physicians in these fields of interest. Therefore, if an insurance company has fulfilled its requirement to provide neurosurgical coverage with *one* "lowest bidder neurosurgeon," even if he or she is board certified, you can be assured that it is inadequate coverage.

WHAT SHOULD HEALTH INSURANCE BE?

Some view health insurance as a prepaid all inclusive plan, which should result in limitless coverage and no out-of-pocket health-care costs, which should be provided by either the government or an employer.

Hopefully, after reading the above sections, I have convinced you that this view is really part of the problem. The above description of health insurance sounds great but is completely unrealistic. By definition, insurance is meant to allow for coverage of some unforeseen tragedy, which hopefully will never be necessary. Consider fire insurance for your home. One recognizes that a fire in the home could result in a terrible and unrecoverable loss, and therefore, one takes out an insurance policy to cover the possible future loss, but never plans on receiving any monetary compensation unless a fire were to occur. The amount of money paid in, over years, is much less than the amount of coverage but still can be a significant amount of money. If investments on the money are made by the insurance company, and interest accumulates, there can be substantial increases realized on the relatively small payments over time. However, the insured never thinks twice about recovering that money after the fact because he is aware that the insurance company was taking the risk for far more than the value of the money paid in premiums. Because many other people are also making payments to protect themselves against an unlikely but devastating fire, enough money accumulates to be able to replace the entire monetary loss of one of the many insured homes if necessary. If people actively pursue decreasing the risk of a fire by installing sprinkler systems and fire alarms, the premiums are reduced because the risk of damages is also reduced.

Car insurance is also similar in that one accepts the responsibility of making payments up front to protect against possible damage to the car or injuries to people in the car in the case of an accident. Premiums are reduced for safe drivers and premiums are increased for those with bad driving records and with histories of prior claims being paid from previous car accidents. When purchasing an automobile, one understands that the price of the car and type of vehicle will have significant influences on the cost of the insurance premiums. Again, no one wants to use the insurance money, because that would mean an accident had occurred, and if used, the cost of future insurance would certainly rise.

For historical reasons, as alluded to in prior chapters, people, for whatever reason, seem to view health insurance in a completely different light than fire or automobile insurance. They seem to think of health insurance as prepaid health dollars, which need to be spent, especially if a deductible has already been met. As I alluded to earlier, I believe that the advent of HMOs had a deleterious effect on promoting this mind-set.

I believe that health insurance should be thought of as a means for a collective group of people to pay into a common pool of funds in order to share the risk of possible future medical needs of individuals within that group. Each will benefit within this group of people who pay into the system by knowing that they will have a certain level of security should such a necessity arise in the future. No single person or group of people within the group should become rich at the expense of others paying into the system. Nonprofit, or mutually self-insured, groups are in my opinion the ideal. Corporate insurance groups with profit motives and executives and shareholders to answer to cannot have the best interest of the client's medical needs at the forefront and therefore should be avoided if possible. If the nonprofit mutual insurance group were able to invest their funds and obtain a substantial collective sum of protection, insurance premiums would go down and costs would be saved. However, if funds are increased in the for-profit corporate model, the excess money is simply siphoned off and given to the rich executives, while the client/potential patients continue to pay high premiums. This model is clearly not ideal for cost savings.

Ideally, it should be possible for relatively large groups of like-minded individuals, such as church groups, unions, or large corporations to be self-insured in such a mutual cost-sharing insurance system. Each member and contributor of such a self-insured group would have voting rights for decisions of what the specifics of care provided would be, such as what level of capitation of maximum output is appropriate, and what is an appropriate deductible. The costs of premiums relative to coverage options and possible discounts relative to health status or additional fees assessed for smoking/obesity, etc., could all be determined by the group. The administrators of the plan would be completely transparent in their costs of administration as would be the financial health of the collective mutually owned insurance company.

MEDICAL RESEARCH

In simple terms, economics plays a large role in medicine today. If Medicare codes related to reimbursement are changed, practice patterns follow and adapt to those changes. There are certain procedures or medical treatments, which are truly believed to be beneficial in certain situations and in highly selected patients but which are currently not covered by insurance companies due to a lack of convincing evidence in the current medical literature. Due to the lack of coverage, these procedures are simply not available. Currently, the pressure to prove efficacy for treatments has been significantly increased by the government compared to times past. The problem is that the clinical research required to prove efficacy and cost-effectiveness of treatment is also very costly and time-consuming. There is currently a difficult conundrum with respect to conducting this type of clinical research. If a new drug or procedure is being considered, the company who develops the new device or pharmaceutical is financially incentivized to fund the research in order to later make a profit, if the research proves positive outcomes. But therein lies a built in conflict. They only want to fund studies and design studies that are likely to succeed on their behalf.

There are serious questions about the results of studies funded in this for-profit model since all involved may be less than honest, even with themselves, about negative results. But even beyond this problem is a concern that much of clinical research that needs to be done has no real tangible profit to be gained as a result of the study. If a relatively straightforward surgical procedure, which does not require new or patented devices, needs to be tested for efficacy in a certain illness, there is no company or entity other than the government to fund the research for the study. Likewise, if a medicine, which has been available for years and is no longer patent protected, is being considered for a novel indication in a relatively rare disease, there is no company willing to fund a research study to prove its efficacy. Well-designed clinical research studies take considerable time, money, and effort to perform.

Institutional review boards (IRBs) are a big part of every major medical center and learning institution. The IRB is a committee that has been formally designated to approve, monitor, and review medical research involving humans. These committees are composed of physicians, nurses, administrators, and even clergy and laypeople. The IRB is responsible for assuring that research is done in an ethical and scientifically sound manner with a great emphasis on protecting the rights of anyone who may be asked to participate in the research. A study must not only be safe, but well thought out and medically justified. Large volumes of paperwork are generated for every proposed project and reviewed by all committee members. This is, of course, very important but time consuming. Involvement in this research process requires a significant dedication and sacrifice of those involved. Some people are employed for the purposes of research directly, however, in many cases, especially physicians, time devoted to research actually takes away from monetarily compensated time spent attending to clinical practice or time in surgery. And as a testament to the scientific dedication of most physicians, many doctors are involved in research in an environment of an actual financial disincentive.

Many universities and larger medical institutions place a significant value on research publications, recognizing an improved status and reputation of the institution, which is gained by the publicity associated with medical publishing. Therefore many, in academic practices, are financially compensated for time spent in research. There are many physicians who are purely researchers and devote all of their time in these endeavors and forgo clinical practice altogether. The financial models of all these factors of compensation for research results vary widely from one institution to another. In most centers, however, the mantra, "publish or perish" is the norm. Furthermore, most academic-related salaries are dependent on obtaining research grants from the government, philanthropic organizations, or venture capitalist business funds in order to continue their work.

Much of scientific discovery in the past has been as a result of serendipity. The discovery of penicillin, as previously discussed, had nothing to due with looking for it. It was discovered by an astute observation of moldy bread. It seems then that by strictly limiting the design of research proposals, we may be decreasing the ability for new groundbreaking discoveries. There needs to remain significant open-ended research opportunities for the purest of scientific reasons, that is, the simple quest for discovery of knowledge without a profit motive. It is generally accepted that much more advancement in science and technology was gained from the space program's endeavor to reach the moon than had been anticipated. We did not simply accomplish the goal of landing a man on the moon. All computer and communication technology was advanced by the "giant step for mankind." My point is simply that another accepted and vital role of government is in the continued support of basic and clinical medical research.

END-OF-LIFE CARE AND "DEATH PANELS"

It has been documented that for most people, the vast majority of funds on health care are expended in the last six months of a person's life. In some sense, this is an obvious and moronic statement, like "people have been found to spend most of their travel money during vacation periods," or "most car accidents have been found to occur within twenty-five miles of a person's home." Obviously, from a statistical point of view, most people drive 90 percent of the time on their way back and forth to their homes and therefore would have an approximate 90 percent chance of having an accident, if one were to occur, happen near their home. Obviously, if someone is an otherwise healthy individual and never went to the hospital and then contracted an illness, which later was determined to be terminal, almost all of the health-care dollars expended in his lifetime will have been spent during the treatment of that terminal illness. Likewise, healthy people involved in traumatic accidents, who die as a result of those accidents, typically have a significant amount of money spent on trying to save their lives before they pass on.

This end-of-life-cost observation has been the topic of significant debate regarding a possible opportunity for health-care savings. Indeed, during the 2008 election debates, this topic was brought up with recommendations of medical expert panels aimed at limiting care expenses, which had been deemed futile. This concept certainly has merit, but it was shot down with a catchphrase label "death panels" championed by Sarah Palin. A cost control panel of fifteen government-appointed and nonelected employees, not necessarily physicians, is included in Obamacare. This panel is seen as threatening and unnerving to many because it places the government between the patient and his or her physician in deciding when to continue or discontinue care.

The idea of diminishing costs of medical interventions at the end of life is, as stated, a viable and important concept. The premise is that if a patient has a terminal condition and no known interventions will have a reasonable chance of extending the life of that patient to any substantial degree, or significantly improving the quality of life for that patient, then these procedures should not be performed. Although simple in principal, this is a very difficult hurdle to jump. It presumes that physicians have a crystal ball and know when a treatment is futile and have certain knowledge of the eventual outcome of the patient. In some cases, this is not too difficult; however, in others, there are significant uncertainties and problems in attempting to predict the future for individual patients. I believe that most, if not all physicians, have been pleasantly surprised by some patients encountered during their careers, which have seemingly beaten the odds and have made remarkable recoveries in spite of multiple serious medical problems, which were life threatening. Even if most patients with similar sets of conditions expire, occasional outliers give us hope on the one hand but cause us to doubt our convictions on the other. I am currently following several patients who are alive and well up to ten years after treatment for a highly malignant brain tumor called a glioblastoma (GBM). The average survival for patients with GBMs, even with current aggressive treatment protocols, is about fifteen months with the vast majority dying before two years and only 1 percent still being alive at five years. Some have suggested that treatment of GBMs is futile. However, if we stop treating all these patients aggressively, those few outliers, who could be cured would never have the chance. Furthermore, by halting aggressive clinical trials and research in this area, we will never make advances for future patients.

The problem is made even more difficult when the physicians feel relatively certain that treatment is futile, but the families or legal representatives of the patient are unwilling to limit or discontinue care due to any number of reasons. Simple ignorance of medical conditions, distrust of the medical professions, alternative belief systems or deep religious convictions of an eventual cure by miracle, and simple denial all become significant barriers to discussing limitations and discontinuation of medical care, even if deemed appropriate by numerous consultants and multidisciplinary medical experts.

The possible cost savings from this type of care restriction or limitation are, in my opinion, enormous. I have taken care of countless numbers of patients in intensive care units over the past twenty-four years. The cost of care in these units is staggering. Single day expenditures of tens of thousands of dollars are the norm and weekly bills of hundreds of thousands of dollars are typical. Often these interventions, including mechanical ventilation and countless intravenous drips of numerous medications and artificial nutritional supplementation, result in the eventual recovery and salvage of life, which would have been unthinkable just one generation prior. However, sometimes, the condition is truly futile and all these heroic efforts are truly in vain (no pun intended) and result in significant unnecessary costs. The trick is to determine ahead of time, which patients may truly benefit from such care and which ones have little or no chance. The current default is to maximally treat all patients until they have either died in spite of all possible interventions or have been determined to have no chance of meaningful survival before discontinuation of care is discussed.

It strikes me as somewhat curious that the default status for every patient entering the hospital regardless of age or overall medical condition is to be a "full code." This means that if an event, such as a cardiac arrest, or other serious life-threatening situation occurs, then an attempt to resuscitate the patient with electric shocks and tubes in every orifice will be performed. I find it almost criminal that a ninety-year-old, who would have otherwise died peacefully at home, when in a hospital environment, will be shocked, chest-pumped, intubated, and placed on mechanical ventilation and catheterized in every orifice before being allowed to expire. Hospital administrators may be financially happy with the status quo however insurance companies and government agencies responsible for paying these bills may have a different point of view.

When individuals contemplate an existence in which they are dependent on others for simple acts of life, like eating and bathing and eliminating biological wastes, almost invariably, say that they would deny themselves of any chance of ending up in such a condition. However, it has been my observation that when those same people are faced with a decision regarding a loved one or family member, they have a very difficult time in making any decision which would cause a limitation of care to prevent their loved one from ending up in such a condition.

It is therefore very important that each of us make these decisions ahead of time for ourselves. In my opinion, these advanced directives, as they are called, need to be somehow on the person and easily available in any emergency condition. It would be best for them to be incorporated electronically into our government-issued identification cards like our drivers licenses. Furthermore, our medical histories and important medical information and medications and medical allergies should be retrievable from our IDs to allow for accurate and timely treatments in any emergency situation. Some have suggested that a subcutaneous silicon chip could easily be implanted with such information, which would allow assurance of all accurate information to be available even if you showed up at the emergency room naked and unconscious. This technology already exists and is quite inexpensive. The amount of time and money saved on every individual would be substantial. Imagine a patient with a known cardiac arrhythmia and EKG abnormality who had a copy of their abnormal EKG electronically available on their person. If that person presented unconscious in a trauma bay after an auto accident, the EKG abnormality would be seen and compared to the prior rhythm in the implanted chip. If the EKG were unchanged, countless money would be saved in avoiding unnecessary additional tests and cardiology consultations. Similarly, brain scans of patients with stable but chronic conditions like hydrocephalus with shunts or brain cysts or benign tumors could be stored on these implanted chips and prevent countless unnecessary additional scans and consultations from being ordered. We will address portability and access of medical information again later. Let's go back to the advanced directives.

In countries like the United Kingdom with socialized medicine, issues of advanced directives may be less important because there are significant restrictions on aggressive care in the elderly. For example, no one over the age of fifty-five receives chronic dialysis for renal failure. There are significant restrictions regarding surgical procedures for those over seventy years of age. In America, however, it is illegal when writing a research protocol to restrict the inclusion of patients into a potential treatment study based on age. It is common for octogenarians to be enrolled in cancer treatment paradigms in America. Age restrictions are frowned upon in America, and it is forbidden to restrict an individual's right for medical treatment based on age. Not all eighty- to ninety-year-olds are equal. I recently ran in the Tucson Marathon and was very impressed to learn of a gentleman at the age of ninety-eight who completed the marathon in six and a half hours. He is likely in superior health and fitness compared to many sixty- to seventy-year-olds. It would be wrong to deny this man care simply based on age. I attended a neurosurgery conference where a case report was presented of a 103-year-old woman who was otherwise healthy and independent but had fallen and developed a large subdural hematoma (blood clot beneath her skull compressing her brain). Somewhat reluctantly on the part of the neurosurgeon, she underwent a craniotomy for removal of her subdural hematoma and remains alive and well seven years later at the age of 110. Conversely, there are many forty- to sixty-year-olds who have abused their bodies with drugs, tobacco, and alcohol for years who have numerous medical conditions, which are now irreversible and avoiding expensive, but futile treatments for them is actually quite reasonable. So who decides which patients are appropriate for treatments and who is responsible for rationing or restricting care to individuals even if they or their families want treatments, which are futile?

I attended a political forum directed by Congressman John Shadegg during the time period before the passage of Obamacare. Congressman Shadegg presented his views on health-care reform to approximately two hundred physicians from numerous subspecialties and backgrounds. There was significant time allotted for comments and questions from the physicians in attendance at this meeting. There seemed to be a great deal of support for this concept of expert medical panels being given the authority to determine when care was futile in order to contain unnecessary costs in end-of-life situations. There were multiple comments made in this setting, which were quite memorable. One such comment went something like this:

An elderly woman referred to as "grandma" was in an intensive care unit (ICU) on mechanical ventilator support for several weeks and making no progress toward recovery. The family insisted on all aggressive care being continued until the insurance policy of one million dollars had been expended. At this point, the hospital financial representative sat down with the family and explained that they would be on the hook for the bill from this time forward. Immediately upon hearing that statement, the family was quoted as saying, "Grandma has put up a good fight, pull the plug."

This anecdote illustrates again the power of economic factors in medical decision-making. When there is no perceived responsibility for payment, people will generally want all tests and procedures performed even with little or no hope for benefit. However, when even small co-payments are required, it can serve as a significant deterrent for accumulating excessive costs. A parking garage attendant informed me of a woman in an expensive Mercedes who complained bitterly of a one-dollar parking charge when she thought the parking was free. I was also told of a person who made a huge scene in a physician's office by screaming and yelling profanities about a twenty-five-dollar co-pay after he had received a quadruple bypass procedure after suffering a heart attack.

I had an experience with an individual in my practice, which brings this point out very clearly. I had implanted a deep-brain-stimulating electrode in this man on a Monday. He was to return for the implant of the necessary internal pulse generator as an outpatient procedure the following Friday morning. Even though he was completely stable and ready for discharge from the hospital on Tuesday morning, he requested to stay in the hospital until Friday because it would save him twenty dollars in cab fare to get back to the hospital. In other words, his government insurance plan had already spent about thirty thousand dollars for his medical procedure, but he thought nothing of them spending another ten thousand dollars or so for an extra three days in the hospital in order for him to save twenty bucks of his own in cab fare. These examples pound home the point that I am trying to make. Unless people share at last some of the responsibility for the costs of their health care and health-care decisions, the costs will never be controlled.

THE COST OF CANCER

Cancer (The big C-word that no one wants to hear) is the number one cause of death in America today. And judging upon the development of numerous cancer centers, there is apparently big money in cancer treatments. Indeed, national chains of cancer centers offering comprehensive and holistic approaches to cancer diagnosis are heavily advertised. Well-established, world-renowned cancer centers like MD Anderson are opening up branch offices in additional locations beyond Texas and advertise their services heavily in these new markets. The good news for those patients diagnosed with cancer today is that people are living longer today than ever before after being diagnosed with cancer and, in some cases, long-term survivors and even cures are becoming more common. However, the bad news for insurance carriers, and the government health-care budget, is that these new diagnostic tests and treatments are extremely expensive.

I treat patients with metastatic tumors to the brain and with malignant primary brain tumors every week. These treatments are very expensive. After surgery, adjunctive radiation and chemotherapy regimens are typically recommended. Some form of chemotherapy is often continued for the remainder of the patient's life. Surveillance MRI scans and PET scans are ordered and performed on a relatively frequent basis in order to monitor the progress of the disease and the effects of the treatments.

One of the relatively new agents for treating brain tumors is an agent called bevacizumab with the trade name Avastin. This agent belongs to a new class of medications called antiangiogenesis drugs. There are numerous other similar drugs in this class currently in clinical trials, which may become available for clinical use in the near future. The sophistication of the science behind the development of these new drugs is truly remarkable but also very expensive. It had been noted for years that tumors are generally more vascular than normal tissue. Obviously, tumor cells, if they are to survive and multiply, require a blood supply to nourish the cells with glucose and oxygen and other nutrients. Molecules and chemical messengers were discovered, which are secreted by cancer cells and which promote vascular proliferation to occur. Avastin and its cousins are molecules, which block or suppress this vascular proliferation in hopes of blocking or suppressing tumor growth. Literally billions of dollars have been spent on the discovery, development, laboratory work and clinical testing of these agents in order to make them available for the fight against cancer.

I know and work with several scientific researchers who are dedicated to understanding cancer cells and discovering the bio molecular properties of these cells, which may prove to be valuable as future anticancer agents to be developed for a possible cure of this disease. I am personally involved in a laboratory research project, which is aimed at discovering how brain cancer cells develop resistance to radiation therapy. It is our hope that by discovering the mechanisms of radiation resistance, we will be able to counteract it and make these cells more vulnerable to radiation treatment, so that the cancer cells won't recur and so that the treatment may be curative for more of our patients. Invariably these scientists are dedicated to this work and are sincere in their desire to discover a cure to these dreaded cancer diseases. Most of them, I don't perceive, even dream of becoming rich or personally gaining from the fruits of their labors, except for the possible prestige in the scientific community of publishing or presenting their work to other colleagues in scientific meetings.

However, the cynic in me has come to the realization that although most are altruistic in this great endeavor of finding a cure for cancer, it has also become big business. Indeed, really big business. Stocks surge with reports of studies confirming positive effects of new anticancer drugs. Patents of new agents are vigorously defended and intellectual property law is a booming business in itself. Conversely, the stocks tumble when negative data as to a drug's effectiveness are published or when serious adverse side effects are reported. Magazine covers have been devoted to so-called "molecules of the year." Literally billions of dollars are at stake financially when it comes to potential cancer cures.

When pharmaceutical companies invest millions, and yes, even billions of dollars in the development of these new agents, they feel justified at charging high prices for the use of these drugs when they finally reach the clinic. I have seen the charges for these drugs from the hospital and the sticker shock is remarkable. The cost of Avastin is over ten thousand dollars per infusion, and these infusions are given typically every two weeks. If a patient does well with this therapy and it is continued for a year, that is twenty-six infusions at a cost of a quarter of a million dollars. Another agent called temozolomide with the trade name Temodar was a major breakthrough several years ago in the treatment of primary brain tumors. It is taken orally, as a simple pill five days per month. Each little pill however is about one thousand dollars. Those five pills would be more than a mortgage payment on a very nice home.

I sometimes implant chemotherapy directly into the brain after I have removed a brain tumor. This is administered in small absorbable dime-sized discs called Gliadel wafers. Each wafer costs about $1,500 and we typically use eight of them at a time. That is an extra twelve thousand dollars for what is reported as an average increase in survival for the patient of an extra six to eight weeks of life compared to similar patients who do not receive these wafers. The phrase "time is money" was never more appropriately stated. What is a week of life worth in dollars? This is a philosophical question for which there is no definite answer.

The most often used catchphrase in medicine today is "quality of life." The issue is however that a high quality of life for one person is not equivalent to that of another. I think we can all agree that a week spent in excellent health in a beautiful beach house with loved ones and family while enjoying leisure activities of swimming, surfing, and sailing would qualify as a high quality of life. Indeed, many of us spend thousands of dollars for vacations in willing pursuit of such quality time. Conversely, an extra week spent in pain, confined to a bed, and unaware of the people around you is not a meaningful existence and money spent to further extend this state of agony is wasted. However, there are many shades of gray between these two extremes.

A patient for whom I cared, for nearly a decade comes to mind. She was a young woman in her thirties who was diagnosed and treated for a highly malignant brain tumor (GBM) more than nine years ago. I was not her original surgeon; I would neither take credit for nor recommend the treatment she was given, even though she had remarkably survived about ten times longer than expected. Her tumor was in her left, dominant hemisphere and therefore affected her ability to speak and use the right side of her body. She was treated with standard radiation therapy after her first surgery but then at recurrence was treated again with another type of radiation called stereotactic radiosurgery. She underwent another surgery several months after this procedure and at the end of this procedure a third type of radiation called brachytherapy seeds were implanted. This triple dose of intense radiation in the brain produced a severe reaction to the brain called radiation necrosis, which literally means dead brain, or, as we speak somewhat callously, brain rot.

I was asked by one of our neuro-oncologists to perform yet another operation on this poor woman due to the severe swelling in her brain, which had caused her to have an inability to speak at all or use the right side of the body. The massive swelling was causing a herniation syndrome where the swollen brain, confined by the skull, spreads over to the other side and compresses the still-functional brain. Due to increased pressure inside the skull, blood flow to normal tissue is limited and this results in brain death unless corrected urgently. At the time, I truly thought the situation was hopeless. I informed her family that even if we did temporarily save her life with another "debulking" surgery, it would not allow her to ever speak or use the right side of the body again. And as is usually the case with this type of tumor, the cancer would likely recur again anyway. I reluctantly agreed to operate again at the insistence of the family and the neuro-oncologist. That was nine years ago. All of the tissue we removed was indeed dead brain but with no viable tumor cells.

Her quality of life was not what I would want, but to her and her family, it was meaningful. After extensive therapy, she could communicate with simple words and phrases and gestures. She wore braces and splints and with assistance proudly stated in clinic that she could sometimes take over one hundred steps in a row. She had to undergo multiple additional surgeries to repair her skin and skull, which were also damaged by the radiation, but it eventually healed. The remarkable thing to me is that she appeared truly happy every time I saw her. She had an amazing crooked smile and with tears said, "Thank you," to me for giving her another chance. I felt a twinge of guilt every time she was so sincerely grateful because I knew that I only did the surgery against my own better judgment.

Recently, this remarkable woman finally passed away after secondary seizures caused by a repeated hemorrhage into the tumor resection bed. Her family anguished with the decision of possibly operating again to remove this blood clot. It was truly uncertain if she had recurrent cancer or not, nearly ten years after her original diagnosis. Her children, now young adults, were tearful but resolute in stating that they would selfishly desire to keep her alive, but they had a conversation with their mother about additional surgery and that she had determined not to have any additional surgeries if the need arose again. There were several anxious and tearful days after withdrawing care before she passed, but all were at peace with this difficult decision.

The point of the above anecdote is to illustrate how very complicated the quality of life problem is and to further explain that even with all the published data and clinical studies we cannot predict outcomes with 100 percent accuracy. If I had not been compelled to operate on this young woman, I would not likely have thought about her again. She would have been the victim of a self-fulfilling prophesy and died as expected from a brain tumor which has less than 1 percent five-year survivorship. I also don't want the reader to misconstrue this outcome as a miraculous recovery with an excellent outcome worth all the effort and cost. I am sure some insurance administrator reading this is cringing at the thought of all the medical bills these extra ten years of life have cost in real dollars. She was by no means functionally or financially independent. She resided in a care center for several years and was visited there frequently by her family. She fortunately had a loving and supportive family and, due to state assistance, was able to obtain the continued medical care that she needed. We can all feel very good about the fact that she had been able to watch her children grow up into mature young adults and enjoy watching and sharing in some of the milestones in the lives of her children. She was a fully conscious and sentient being up to the last few days of her life and felt that her life is worth living, and maybe that is all that matters.

A very famous example of someone with a limited quality of life from an external point of view is the astrophysicist Steven Hawking, who amazingly continues to survive in spite of the fatal Lou Gherig's disease, also known as amyotrophic lateral sclerosis (ALS) he was inflicted with. It is doubtful that anyone else with his extent of disease would still be alive, but due to his resources, and obvious will to live, he has continued to survive and be productive in his research and writing. I am personally a big fan of his and am grateful that he is still with us, but I must admit that if I were in his circumstances, I don't know if I would wish to continue living the way he does. His case brings home two points I am trying to make. One is that quality of life is a very subjective and personal matter, which is impossible to make clear and concise measurements on. The second is that, as medical science advances, there will be more and more patients in difficult situations, which may be able to have their lives extended, but at great monetary costs. The real question is, who will be responsible for bearing those costs, and who will decide which patients are entitled to such resources if they do not possess them on their own? I propose that these costs will be far too high for all who may wish to use these resources to be able to receive them. Can we really afford to supply every aging and immobile person in America with a computer-assisted scooter?

That is really the crux of the problem we are facing in this big medical economics mess we are in right now. The medical technologies we have developed are far more complicated and much more expensive than in the past. Due to the aging population, and the existence of increasing numbers of patients with aging-related diseases such as cancer, the real monetary costs will continue to escalate simply due to the sheer numbers of treatments needed. Ironically, successful treatments, which extend life, will only further escalate the costs. As the percentage of people over the age of sixty-five continues to expand out of proportion to those in the working and productive years between the ages twenty to sixty-five, it will become increasingly burdensome for the working population to subsidize and support the medical care of the elderly population. It really is that simple, if not depressing, to face this harsh reality. I liken it to the current situation in Greece. The GNP of Greece does not match the amount of money previously allocated to retirement entitlements and is therefore insolvent. Our Medicare and state-sponsored Medicaid plans are also soon to be insolvent based on projections of the aging population and rising costs of medicine. Unless we face this harsh reality, we will face similar austerity measures that have brought the Greek citizens to riot in the streets.

THE COST OF MEDICAL DEVISES AND PHARMACEUTICALS

$\bigwedge\!\!\bigwedge\!\!\bigwedge\!\!\bigwedge$

I will now address the issue of the excessive costs of medications and the outlandish prices of medically implanted devices. It is estimated that it costs approximately one billion dollars to bring a new drug to market. That is a staggering amount of money when one considers that the actual chemical may be relatively simple to produce and may even be a natural substance. In many cases, pharmaceuticals are slightly modified molecules based on naturally occurring chemical compounds with a discovered medicinal value. Many antibiotics are based on chemicals produced naturally by fungi, which allow them to grow in the presence of bacteria, by either killing the bacteria or limiting the bacteria's ability to grow.

The discovery of penicillin from common bread mold is the most famous example of this and has had an unbelievable effect on our ability to treat infectious diseases. Penicillin of course is actually dirt cheap to produce but, unfortunately, today has limited application because of the development of resistant strains of bacteria, which have arisen. Scientists have developed ingenious ways to modify these naturally occurring antibiotics in order to still allow them to be useful and to subvert the bacteria's means of resistance. Research and development continues to be employed by major pharmaceutical companies in hopes of finding new and hopefully more effective antibiotics or new ways of modifying existing ones to make them safer or more efficacious against these resistant strains of bacteria. But having a few chemists playing around in a lab and test for efficacy of modified substances against some bacteria in petri dishes and test tubes does not cost a billion dollars. Research grants for elaborate brain tumor research, of which I am partially involved, are in the range of hundreds of thousands of dollars and allow for the discovery of some exciting new compounds in the fight against brain cancer. The largest grants of one to five million dollars are celebrated by research scientists and their institutions and go a long way for helping in the fight against this terrible monster: cancer. And again, a million dollars is only 1/1000th of a billion. Why such a great cost to bring new agents into the clinical arena?

I propose that a very large component of the cost of medicines is to be blamed on the litigious environment in which we live. Again, watch daytime TV for any amount of time at all, and you will be solicited to join in a class action suit with promises of possible financial compensation for side effects caused by any number of currently or recently available medications or devices. The federal drug administration (FDA) requires extensive, and some would say excessive, safety and efficacy testing to be performed prior to the release of any new drug. These tests are initially performed on laboratory animals for sometimes years prior to ever allowing use in humans. If these tests are accomplished without any signs of toxicity, then tightly controlled phase 1, 2, and 3 human trials are allowed to occur. Phase 3 trials are randomized, placebo-controlled trials with strictly defined safety and efficacy outcome measures in large enough cohorts of patients to assure the drug is of clinical value and has an acceptable safety profile. These trials typically take a few years to complete and of course may result in a negative result, thus costing the sponsoring company millions of dollars in the process without any fruit to bear. Even if the results are positive and the drug is released to the market, there are costs of marketing and sales and distribution as with any business. The major liability risks, however, do not occur until after the drug is released for clinical use.

During the testing process, typically a few thousand or even tens of thousands of people may be exposed to the effects of the medications in clinical trials. But some side effects, especially the most dangerous idiosyncratic reactions, may not become apparent until hundreds of thousands or millions of patients are treated with medications. Typically in clinical trials, the patients who are enrolled have well defined conditions and are screened for other possible confounding medical conditions in order to be included in the studies. However, when the new medication is released to the market in the real world, all types of patients, who may be taking numerous other medications with possible serious drug interactions are exposed to the new compounds. It takes numerous observant physicians with the willingness to investigate and report untoward effects of new medications before previously unforeseen side effects or even lethal reactions become apparent. The saga of the selective COX-2 inhibitors described earlier illustrates this point.

A current example involves a new class of drugs, which are used as anticoagulants (blood thinners in layman's terms) as an alternative to Coumadin. Coumadin is an old and cheap drug, which is actually a component of rat poison. This medication is a liver toxin for humans as well, and because the liver produces the coagulation factors for the blood, by poisoning the liver, people on this medication do not produce normal amounts of clotting factors, and the desired therapeutic effect of anticoagulation is achieved. For years, people have been treated with Coumadin for several clinical conditions in which diminishing the blood's tendency to clot is desirable. The most common indications are for people with deep venous thrombosis (DVTs), which are large clots, usually in the deep central veins in the legs, and atrial fibrillation, which is an abnormal rhythm in the heart. Both of these conditions are life threatening. People with DVTs can have a portion of the clot break of in the legs and travel into the heart and lungs and cause death by lack of blood flow and oxygenation by blocking the heart and lungs. People with atrial fibrillation have a tendency to form clots in the upper chambers of the heart due to a lack of effecting pumping action caused by this condition. These clots can then migrate to the lungs and cause poor oxygenation or to the brain and cause strokes.

There is good reason for all of us to have clotting factors in our blood, that is, to keep us from bleeding to death if we are cut or injured. There is a constant and fine-tuned balancing act in all of us between clot formation and clot dissolution. Physicians understand that by giving anticoagulants like Coumadin, they are tipping the scale away from clot formation and toward clot dissolution. People on Coumadin are at a known increased risk of bleeding and this can be life threatening. Nearly all people on Coumadin bruise more easily because a bruise is really a small amount of blood extravasated out under the skin.

One of the major challenges of neurosurgery (some would say, "The bane of our existence") is to treat people on Coumadin with bleeds into their brains. It actually seems to be the norm rather than the exception to encounter patients with Coumadin-related brain hemorrhages every time I am on call. A simple bump on the head for someone on Coumadin, many times not even remembered by the patient or family, can result in the accumulation of blood over the surface of the brain because a tiny capillary tear, which simply continues to ooze into this space without the normally active clotting factors available to stop it. This extravasated blood forms into a large subdural hematoma and can compress the brain and cause seizures or weakness or even death. In order to perform life-saving surgery for these patients, the anticoagulation effects must be reversed before surgery, or else they would bleed to death on the table. Recurrence of the subdural hematomas happens way more often than we would like. I have often wondered if the risks of Coumadin are worth the benefits because of the number and the severity of the problems with this drug that we encounter. Of course, all of this has been well studied, and the results are in favor of treatment with Coumadin for correctly selected patients; however, the risks and side effects of treatment are very real with about seven intracranial bleeds per year per one thousand patients on Coumadin.

It is important to understand that these serious side effects of anticoagulation are well understood and can never be completely eliminated. It is important for patients on Coumadin to be frequently monitored with blood tests to assure that the level of anticoagulation remains within the therapeutic range and is not excessive. Coumadin also has several interactions with other drugs that are metabolized in the liver that can make adjustments to medication levels very challenging. Because of the many difficulties in managing patients on Coumadin, there have been several new agents developed as alternatives. Pradaxa (Dabigatran) is the most prominent of these new agents.

Pradaxa does not require frequent blood tests for monitoring and was found to reduce the number of intracranial hemorrhages by two-thirds in one international study of eighteen thousand patients compared to Coumadin. It was also superior in diminishing the number of strokes for patients with atrial fibrillation by 34 percent compared to Coumadin but did have a higher incidence of stomach bleeding. This new direct thrombin inhibitor is considered a great advance even though it is much more expensive ($3.20 per day compared to $0.40 per day) because of the advantages as described above.

These superior results however did not inhibit the lawyers from developing a class action lawsuit against this drug. There are currently daily TV ads for 1800-BAD-Drug promising compensation for users of this drug because of the occurrence of brain hemorrhages. There are about five other new similar agents in the class of direct Thrombin inhibitors, which may even be better alternatives; however, these have not been as well studied.

My point is that the cost of this drug is already high due to product liability. If more and more lawsuits are won or waged against this and other similar new drugs, the costs will become prohibitive. Or worse, some of these agents may never reach the market or will be discontinued due to the costs of defending the suits. Isn't it interesting that there are no class action lawsuits against Coumadin even though it has a higher bleeding risk? I assume that is because there is no money in generic drugs for the lawyers to go after. Isn't it an ironic travesty that more people could have unnecessary bleeds into their brains on Coumadin instead of being on newer, safer drugs because of the lawyers who are supposedly protecting us from these bad drugs?

Several of my colleagues perform complex spine operations on a daily basis. They typically implant titanium screws and rods into the spine for stabilization and reconstruction for patients who would otherwise have an unstable spine. I find it alarming that the hospital charges for these screws implanted into the spine are typically several hundred dollars each. More complex hardware such as expandable cages and plating fixation devices cost several thousand dollars each. If you go to Home Depot and look in the hardware department, you can find similar hardware devices which are priced from pennies to a few dollars. Sure, there are quality assurance issues and sterilization processes, which make medical devices more expensive; however, they are clearly not orders of magnitude more expensive to produce when compared to standard hardware items.

I will credit one of my golf buddies Bob, who is a pilot, with this related example. In the 1960s, if you wanted to buy a Cessna personal aircraft, the price was in the same ballpark as an expensive luxury automobile. The list price of a Cessna 172 Skyhawk, when it was first introduced in 1956, was $8,700. By comparison, a 1956 Cadillac was about $5,000. In fact, in 1957, a special production Cadillac Brougham had a price tag of $13,000. In other words, in the 1950s and '60s, the ability to purchase a personal aircraft was within financial reach of a significant portion of the general population. The current price of a Cessna 172 is over $300,000, which is thirty-five times the cost in 1956 and is clearly out of the reach of all except the most wealthy Americans. Median income over the same time period increased by approximately a factor of seven, and the price of luxury cars have increased by approximately a factor of ten. Why did the cost of aircraft escalate so much more than luxury automobiles and standard inflation over the same time period?

In the sixties and seventies, it was quite common for physicians and other professionals to own personal aircraft. It has been speculated that physicians thought they were better pilots than they actually were. If a physician died in a plane crash, crafty lawyers would place part of the blame of the crash on the aircraft's faulty design or equipment or some other malfunction. The survivors would then become the recipients of large monetary awards including compensation for lost income. These lost income payouts could be quite substantial if a prominent cardiologist for example had a high six, or even a seven-figure income. Therefore the product liability component of personal aircraft has made these items so expensive that they are out of reach for the vast majority of people. If these airplanes were less expensive, more people would be able to fly them, and there would be a higher number of jobs in the manufacturing and servicing of small personal aircraft. This is another example of how lawsuit abuse is stifling the American economy in general and not just the field of medicine.

In the field of medicine, and particularly with respect to implantable devices, the highest component of the price can be linked to the product liability. Simply watch any daytime TV show, and you will be inundated with advertisements for claims of compensation relative to surgically implanted devices. All of us are paying for the price of this product liability component in our health insurance premiums and hospital bills. I have been informed that the total bills for spinal fusion procedures for the nation last year was forty-six billion dollars. That is approximately one-thirtieth of the cost of all health-care delivery in the United States combined and is approximately 0.5 percent of the entire gross national product. The exorbitant prices of these products, with a large component being attributed to product liability, can truly bankrupt our country if something is not done.

GOVERNMENT HEALTH CARE

I am tempted to quote President Reagan and state that government is not the solution to the health-care problem but rather government is the problem. However, it is not quite so simple when one considers all that is involved in the administration of health care in a diverse country like America with over three hundred million people. Health care is the most government-regulated industry in the country, and certainly, some regulation is necessary but so much regulation can be stifling. Many, of the more liberal mind-set, have suggested that our government should completely overtake health care and that it would be a great public service. For anyone, like myself, who has spent any amount of time working in a VA (Veteran's Administration) hospital, the idea of this type of medicine is almost unthinkable. Everything runs slowly, inefficiently, and seems bogged down in regulatory red tape and protocols. Most bothersome is the apparent mind-set of many of the employees. As in all aspects of life, generalizations are often overstated and fail to recognize individuals within a group who are exceptional. However, in my experience, many VA hospital employees seemed more concerned with the end of their shift and defining what aspects of the work were *not* in their job description, then about providing compassionate care or improving the system. When trying to get another surgery on the schedule, the usual response was to explain all the reasons why it could not be done that day rather than trying to adjust and adapt and possibly put in extra effort or work overtime. Applications for new equipment needed to be submitted and sent to committees to be preapproved, and then funds would be appropriated seemingly years before it ever would be available for actual use. Sometimes the equipment, by the time it arrived, was already obsolete and needed the next generation to be ordered before it was even in use. In short, working in a purely government-controlled health-care environment was extremely frustrating.

Private sector hospitals have an obvious focus on patient-centered care with an absolute realization that the patient-customer has a choice of where to go for care and will choose the hospital down the street if their experience is not a positive one. The employees—including nurses, transport staff, ward clerks, and service department staffs—are generally more friendly, efficient, and motivated to deliver exemplary service and compassionate patient care. New technologies are seemingly easily obtained and adapted into use on a regular basis. Nearly all private hospitals currently have nicely decorated and medically efficient private rooms, even in an intensive care setting. Whereas government-run hospitals, such as in the VA or Indian Health

System, there remains multibed hospital rooms with less than state-of-the-art equipment with stark industrial style decor. Given the stark contrast, no one in their right mind, when given the choice, would chose to go to a typical VA hospital for their medical care over a modern private hospital. This is much more than an issue of cosmetics and aesthetics. The technology, efficiency, and quality of government run health care are inferior to that provided in the private setting.

It seems to be an unavoidable consequence of human nature that people work better, and are more productive, in a competitive environment where there are tangible incentives for advancement, based on work performance. Conversely, people in a regimented and top-down regulated environment, where only time needs to go by before the next scheduled advancement, and with minimal incentive for change, people seem to do the minimal required amount of work. Individual accountability, responsibility, and opportunity for advancement are optimal or even necessary for productivity in any business, including the business of medicine.

Many more socialized countries have completely government-controlled health care. Our closest neighbor, Canada, has such a system; and numerous comparisons have been made to our system, some positive and some negative. I certainly do not consider myself an expert on the Canadian system; however, we have had several fellows in our program who have come from Canada, and I have had occasion to inquire from those who have actually worked within their system. In many aspects, the system seems to function adequately for many people; however, there are some major problems, which cannot be overlooked. As in the HMO scenario, numerous simple public health functions, like vaccinations and pediatric wellness checks are likely quite superior in their administration compared to our haphazard approach. However, the major complaint has been in regards to the typical waiting periods for surgical or technical procedures. In other words, when you really need a treatment, be prepared to wait. I personally have treated many patients from Canada over the years who have fortunately had the means to come across the border and pay for their brain tumor to be removed here rather than waiting the six to twelve months before it would have been done in Canada.

One of my best friends and golf buddies is from Canada. On one occasion, he invited his cousin, who was visiting from Alberta to join us. He was an otherwise active and healthy man in his forties. I noticed that he walked with a limp, and I asked him what had caused the weakness in one of his legs. He informed me that he had a herniated disc in his back, which had pinched a nerve and caused permanent weakness in his ability to raise his foot. This is a very common sign of an L4-5 herniated disc causing an L-5 radiculopathy, which results in damage to the nerves, which control the muscles, which allow one to raise his foot and extend his great toe. He told me that he had this visible weakness from the beginning of his symptom onset and that it had taken months to get an MRI in Canada, and then another nine months before he had the appropriate surgery to remove the disc and decompress the affected nerve root. So altogether, a year had gone by before he had received the appropriate treatment, and as a result, he had permanent nerve damage and walked with a limp. In our country, it would be considered malpractice to not operate on such a patient within a few days. I have personally operated on several such cases within twenty-four hours of the initial symptom onset because of the fear of permanent nerve damage if not dealt with promptly. I have heard of waiting lists for breast biopsies of nine to twelve months after suspicious mammograms. Obviously, if cancer were present at the time of the positive mammogram, one year later, the cancer could have progressed from a curable stage 1 condition initially to an incurable widespread stage 4 disease state over that time period.

It is an interesting fact that there are more MRI scanners in Maricopa County servicing approximately four million people than there are in the entire country of Canada, which has nearly ten times as many people. I am the director of our Gamma Knife facility, which is one of about 150 Gamma Knives in the United States. The Gamma Knife is a remarkable machine developed by Dr. Lars Leksell in Sweden. This device was the first developed instrument to perform radiosurgery. Radiosurgery is the process of using multiple highly focused and computer-directed gamma rays or X-rays to target and treat a brain tumor or other specific abnormalities in the brain without the need for any opening of the skull. Radiosurgery has literally changed the way that many brain tumors are treated and has significantly diminished pain and suffering for many patients who would otherwise have to undergo open operations. Many of the patients that we treat with the gamma knife really have no other option for treatment, due to the dangerous location within their brain, which would make an open operation extremely risky. Up until a few years ago, Canada did not have a single Gamma Knife, and now they have two for the entire country. Clearly, free market pressures are a much more equitable and efficient means of distributing advanced medical devices compared to government-run bureaucracies.

Several of our residents have gone to Australia to learn from an exceptional surgeon in Sydney. They have informed me of their experiences there, after spending six months in that environment. Australia also has government-run health care, but it is completely accepted as a two-tier system. There is a basic level of health care administered by the Australian government for all citizens who cannot afford more, or who choose not to spend more for private care. It has been described as a no-frills, bare-bones medical system with reasonable care, but with limitations and restrictions and suboptimal wait times. Those who have the means purchase private insurance to allow them to be treated by the physicians of their choice in a more timely manner. Our residents in training would operate with near complete autonomy on patients within the public system hospitals, whereas they would act as assistants and observers to the established surgeons on the private-pay patients in the private hospitals. It seems that both groups of patients were grateful and comfortable with the two-tier system. Those in the public system were generally grateful for the low-cost medicine they received and were grateful for the care they received. Those in the private-pay group felt the increased cost was more than justified and appreciated the increased service and treatment opportunities they received for the extra costs.

So what should the role of the US government in medicine be? The short answer, based on the above-described observations, should be an adequate one to provide care for those in need, but not to overtake the entire system. In reality, providing some degree of medical services for those in need and regulating health care for the country is an appropriate role of government. Providing health care for those who would never be able to afford care is an admirable goal. The difficult task is to decide, define, and limit the scope of government-sponsored care only to those who are truly in need and cannot be responsible financially for their own care.

I have a soft spot in my heart for one group of patients in this category, which I feel are fairly easy to discern as needing government assistance. These are patients with medically refractory epilepsy. Epilepsy affects patients with multiple brain disorders and is more appropriately considered a symptom of an underlying disease rather than a specific entity in and of itself. There are many different types of seizures, ranging from simple partial seizures — where the patient experiences an involuntary aura such as an episode of déjà vu accompanied by a strange smell or taste, but not affecting consciousness — to major convulsions called generalized tonic-clonic or Grand Mal seizures.

Seizures are involuntary and result from many different brain abnormalities, which cause abnormal synchronization of neuronal firing patterns and recruitment of otherwise normal neurons, in a kind of electrical brainstorm. Some patients with epilepsy, which means repeated seizures, have entirely normal appearing brains on MRI scans. These patients usually have an underlying microscopic biochemical abnormality, which causes a susceptibility to seizures. Other patients with epilepsy have grossly abnormal brains, sometimes with large areas of abnormalities affecting one or both hemispheres.

In patients with one obviously abnormal hemisphere, which is entirely dysfunctional and is determined to be the source of their seizures, hemispherectomy is recommended. The removal, or complete disconnection of the affected hemisphere in properly selected patients, has a 90 percent success rate of completely eliminating seizures in these patients. Remarkably, since these patients were born with the abnormal hemisphere, and due to the phenomenon of neuroplasticity, the contralateral normal hemisphere is able to assimilate and accommodate for many of the functions of the missing hemisphere. These patients can typically walk, but they have a mild limp and one hand that is spastic and only partially useful. However, they can have essentially normal speech and intelligence.

I operated on one such patient about ten years ago and disconnected her left hemisphere, which had been injured prior to birth. She unfortunately suffered severe seizures and was considered disabled until the operation was performed at age seventeen. However, after the procedure, she has never had another seizure and is no longer taking any antiepileptic medications. The most amazing result however is that she has since graduated cum laude from a major university and is working as a teacher and has gotten married since the surgery. This case is an example of someone with literally half a brain functioning better than most with both intact cerebral hemispheres. Her case further illustrates how modern medical intervention can dramatically affect someone's life for the better and result in a person becoming financially and socially independent, whereas prior to the intervention, they were completely disabled and dependent on others for all aspects of life, financially and otherwise.

The most common procedure for medically refractory epilepsy is the removal of part of the temporal lobe for patients with a disease called mesial temporal sclerosis (MTS). MTS can result from many different insults to the brain such as trauma or infection or an episode of hypoxia, such as may occur in a near drowning. The most typical scenario is when an infant has a high fever and this causes a febrile seizure. This is fairly common, but if the fever is very high and the seizure is somewhat prolonged, permanent damage to a specialized part of the brain called the hippocampus results.

The hippocampus resides in the medial part of each temporal lobe and is responsible for forming all memories. This small structure is highly metabolically active as it continually files and consolidates each moment in our lives to be retrieved later in a condensed or abstracted form. It is indeed amazing that this part of the brain allows us to form a nearly continuous memory stream of our entire lives. The details of how this hippocampal structure accomplishes this remarkable function are not well understood and are the topics of active research. It is presumed that because of this high metabolic activity, the hippocampus is more vulnerable to states of hypoxia or high fever. It was recently discovered that the hippocampus can actually grow new neurons, even into adulthood. However, these new neurons and sprouting from injured areas probably result in abnormal connections and synchronization of electrical signals, producing seizures, which are particularly difficult to control with medicine. Fortunately, because there are two hippocampi and one is sufficient for memory function, removal of a single injured hippocampus is a highly successful operation and can cure properly selected patients with this disease about 80 percent of the time.

From a financial and social economic standpoint, the procedure of temporal lobe surgery for the cure of epilepsy has been shown to be the most cost effective surgical procedure ever studied. This is because prior to the surgery, patients are often unable to work or be functionally independent and typically spend a significant amount of health-care dollars on anticonvulsant medications and frequent emergency room visits. They sometimes have significant traumatic injuries secondary to the epilepsy, which further adds to the health-care costs. After surgery, especially if they are completely cured, they can be completely functionally independent, wean off of anticonvulsant medications, become gainfully employed, and actually pay taxes. It is estimated that although the preoperative workup and surgery are quite expensive for these patients with temporal lobe epilepsy, the procedure can pay for itself in two to three years. I have given this relatively lengthy example to show that government-assisted coverage for patients who otherwise would not be able to afford their own care is both necessary and even profitable in some instances.

Unfortunately, there are many other situations, particularly in children with severe neurological congenital and traumatic abnormalities in which there is no hope for cure, and for whom, there is no good financial outcome possible. These patients and their families, in the vast majority of cases, would never be able to afford adequate care without government assistance.

Another very difficult and unfortunate group patients are those with mental illness. Schizophrenia is much more common than most people realize. It affects approximately one out of every two hundred people, meaning that approximately 1,500,000 Americans suffer from this disease to some extent. The popular and very well done movie *A Beautiful Mind* personalized this condition for most of us. The hallmark of the disease is the presence of auditory hallucinations and abnormal thoughts injected into one's normal thought processes, which makes the determination of what is real and what is not real very difficult to discern for affected individuals. Unfortunately, the percentage of homeless people who suffer from schizophrenia is remarkably high. These people find it very difficult to maintain employment and fit into society. Many of these people can be quite functional if given a correct diagnosis and adequate medical management and psychiatric counseling. However, due to paranoia and odd behavior, they can be marginalized from society and never seek out proper medical attention. Again, a schizophrenic person, who is homeless and a frequent flyer to emergency rooms can be a significant challenge to the medical system physically and financially. If diagnosed early and properly treated, the same individual could be highly functional and employable. It would behoove us as a nation and as individual states to do a much better job at caring for those with schizophrenia and other challenging mental disorders than we are currently doing.

It is certainly an admirable goal of an advanced society to care for the poor and needy and less fortunate. Those who are sick or suffering, especially due to no fault of their own, should certainly strike a powerful cord in the hearts of all conscientious people. The collective/government-administered programs should be well coordinated to aid in the efforts of alleviating suffering of the poor and afflicted. The challenge again is to determine which patients and families are deserving of complete assistance by the remainder of society and which patients should be held responsible for their own care financially. For example, is it fair for society in general to assume the complete financial burden of an otherwise healthy thirty-year-old who decided to ride a motorcycle recklessly without wearing a helmet and becomes a vegetative survivor? I have heard many motorcycle riders in Arizona, where there is no helmet law, explain that it would be a violation of their personal rights to be forced to wear a helmet. The claim to individual freedom is fine until one considers that I currently have no freedom to choose if my tax dollars help subsidize their care in the current system, when they suffer an incapacitating head injury, which is not severe enough to kill them, but results in them becoming a chronic vegetative survivor in an extended care facility.

Is it fair for society in general to pay for the consequences of smoking-induced lung cancer, emphysema and cardiovascular disease? If someone wants the freedom to enjoy smoking, they must also accept the responsibility of that choice and not force the medical consequences on the rest of us as a great financial burden. Is it fair for society in general to pay for the multiple medical problems accumulated in an individual secondary to obesity? Obese patients have higher risks of cardiac disease, stroke, diabetes, chronic inflammation, and have higher infection rates and overall higher complication rates from all surgical procedures compared to patients with normal body weight. In all other aspects of life, people are responsible for the consequences of their own decisions, but why not in medicine and health care? There has to be some real aspect of personal responsibility in a financially meaningful way in order to curb the cost of health care.

It is not reasonable to believe that helping those who are less fortunate would result in the attainment of equal status or an equivalent level of service. For example, those who have trouble financially can be given food stamps, bus passes, and government-subsidized housing. But they cannot be given mansions in the Hamptons, chauffeur-driven limousines, and personal gourmet chefs.

In the current health-care situation, once someone on Medicaid begins receiving care, they are expected to receive the same level of care and service as those who are insured privately. Furthermore, someone who comes to the emergency room without insurance, and even without being a citizen of the United States, cannot be denied care and has the ability and right to sue for malpractice, without ever spending a dime, or anticipating ever spending a dime of their personal money for their care.

The Boston Tea Party was about taxation without representation. What about the opposite situation, in which there exists a right to litigation without any compensation? Can you go to a rental car company and demand that a car be provided for you and maintain the ability to sue for malfunction of that car without ever paying for the rental of the car? I think not! It is simply not reasonable that someone can receive work/services/time/effort from someone else and expect to pay nothing for it, and possibly have lottery winnings in the form of a malpractice lawsuit if the services are felt to be inadequate.

Physicians are in general very caring and generous people. I know of many physicians who annually go to third world countries to provide services to the poor and needy without any expectation of compensation. They take with them donated goods and equipment from the United States to help the poor with their medical needs, which could not be provided for in their native countries. These physicians find these donated personal services greatly rewarding and even somewhat spiritual in nature. Many comment on the relative ease of giving treatment in these environments with a lack of painstaking documentation to protect themselves from possible lawsuits. How refreshing it is to simply care for people on a one-on-one basis, without fear of litigation! It is a sad reality that although there are many underprivileged neighborhoods in the United States, which could benefit from similar programs, physicians are cautioned not to provide the services here because of the possibility of malpractice lawsuits.

HEALTH-CARE ECONOMICS

In the simplest understanding of economics, money is used as an exchange medium for the intrinsic value of goods and services. Every person will evaluate the value of specific goods or services to themselves personally, and based on that item's assigned monetary cost, that person will determine if that cost is justified enough to utilize their own funds to purchase the item or pay for the service. If the purchase price is deemed too high, relative to that persons means, he will make a conscious decision to forgo the purchase or to perform the desired service for himself.

When I was sixteen, I had worked already for several years in my father's sign business and had been able to save enough money to purchase my own sports car. My pre-owned Triumph TR7 was my pride and joy. Since I had the skills and the painting facilities in my father's shop, I painted it myself in Dupont's newest paint, Imron metallic black. I used my own skills to put real gold-leaf pin-stripes and a self-designed logo on the hood to further customize it. I bought Mag wheels and TA radial tires after working extra hours and felt great about each of these purchases when I proudly cruised around Reno in my car. Since it was all my own hard-earned money, I was quite budget conscious, and so I performed all the minor service and oil changes myself. At this time, in the late 1970s, a new service was introduced, drive-through oil changing stations. I still remember the amazement I felt after the first time I went to JiffyLube. It cost only twenty dollars and took only fifteen minutes. I determined then that those twenty dollars were very well spent because for those twenty dollars, someone else did the work to provide the oil and the filter and to spare me the time and hassle of getting under the car and getting all greasy by doing it myself.

Conversely, Home Depot has turned do-it-yourself home projects into a multibillion dollar company. People determine each day what goods and what services they are willing to pay for based on the value of those items or services to them personally, relative to their personal financial situation. Now, because I make a good income as a neurosurgeon, I typically pay for others to perform work and home improvements around my house, but as a resident, that was not the case. On one of my weekends off, I set out to repair my broken garage door. This was a bad decision. The very powerful spring, which provides the lift of the door was unleashed and nearly tore off my right thumb. I had to go to the emergency room and receive stitches. My residency chairman lectured me on the importance of protecting my hands and of my future earning potential. How silly it was to attempt to save a couple hundred bucks at a risk of possibly ruining my future career.

One of the major problems of health-care economics has been the development of the disconnection of realistic monetary values of the medical services provided. Certainly laypeople do not have the option of performing their own brain surgery. But many people do forgo seeing their doctor and self prescribe countless herbal remedies, untested and unproven as they may be, in order to save money by not going to their doctor.

Health care is not free! The amount of hard work and effort involved in obtaining the knowledge and skill to practice medicine in the sophisticated medical environment of the United States is staggering. No other vocation requires more education and time of preparation. It takes fifteen years of schooling, including a seven-year residency to become a neurosurgeon. Many neurosurgeons take an additional year or two in a fellowship for subspecialty training after completing their residency. During my residency, I typically worked well over one hundred hours per week and had very little sleep. In my worst year, as a junior resident, there were months in which I took call every other night. That meant to start work on one day rounding before 5:00 a.m., working all day in the intensive care units (ICUs) and hospital wards, then staying up all night in the emergency room, or ICUs, and then working a normal day thereafter, and then finally leaving the hospital around 7:00–8:00 p.m. I would then go home and briefly see my wife and kids, many times falling asleep in my plate at the dinner table, only to wake up again the next day at 4:30 a.m. to start another forty-hour shift. Yes, that's right, work forty hours, off for eight hours, indefinitely repeated, with only one weekend off per month. In some months, we had a rotating general surgery resident on the service taking calls so that my co-resident and I could take call every third night. This was greatly appreciated, and certainly helped, but on that middle day between calls, I still worked a twelve-to-sixteen-hour shift. I learned an incredible amount that year, and amazingly, I survived my residency and came to realize that the human body has an unbelievable capacity to adapt to extremes of stress and sleep deprivation.

As opposed to President Obama's notions, I did that! No one else did it for me. I will never forget it, and my wife and family suffered along with me. I remember being physically, mentally, and emotionally exhausted and numb. Once, during this time, we went on a one-week vacation to visit my wife's family in California. After four to five days of catching up on sleep and just vegetating on the beach, I began to come out of my fog and remembered what it felt like to feel normal again, enjoying life and feeling close again to those I love. Now, there have fortunately been laws passed against this type of work schedule for residents. They are no longer allowed to work more than eighty hours in a week and not more than twenty-four consecutive hours. I personally believe this is a great change and a necessary change; however, we resident educators are concerned that, with these restricted hours, there may not be enough time and experience to gain all of the knowledge and skills necessary to be a fully trained, independently functioning neurosurgeon.

What is the intrinsic value of an operation performed by a highly trained specialist? What dollar amount is appropriately assigned to reflect the intrinsic value of a procedure performed with this degree of technical expertise? How much is it worth to save a life or diminish pain and suffering? How do you place a value on knowledge and experience and compassion? I suggest simply that there is a significant intrinsic value of medical knowledge and surgical procedures which is very real and tangible and cannot simply be assumed as being free.

The cost of medical education is also staggering. Many practicing physicians enter their careers after investing eleven to seventeen years of time along with a real monetary debt typically in excess of two hundred thousand dollars. These loans and the cumulative interest need to be repaid. There are the tangible overhead costs of the practice of medicine. Office space and examining rooms, office personnel, and nurses all come at a significant expense. As alluded to earlier, malpractice insurance is a significant cost. Neurosurgeons and obstetricians typically spend over one hundred thousand dollars per year for malpractice insurance in most states. All of these costs have to be included in patient billing and add to the relative monetary value of physician services compared to other services economically.

I've spoken nothing the medical equipment required for today's modern procedures. The intraoperative microscope, which I utilize for performing brain surgeries, is a fantastic piece of equipment. It has a balancing system to allow the head of the microscope to float in the air for me to control it's position with an adjustable mouthpiece. This allows me to keep both of my hands free to perform the surgery. I also adjust the focus and magnification levels of the microscope with my mouthpiece and foot pedals. There is a specialized chair designed to integrate with the microscope, which has movable and adjustable arm rests and foot pedals to raise and adjust the height of the chair relative to the microscope and the patient. The microscope today is also equipped with an integrated navigational system, which is registered to each individual patient based on a preoperative MRI scan. This is similar to a global positioning system in your car. The microscope utilizes a high-powered computer connected to a tracking camera device on the microscope, which can simultaneously update my position within the brain including trajectory views along my line of site three-dimensionally. Convergent laser pointers continuously convey to me the focal point of the microscope as it is associated with these trajectory and positional views on the high definition video screens adjacent to the patient in the operating room. Each one of these fantastic microscopes cost around one million US dollars. The MRI scanners used to provide the imaging sets for the navigation to occur and to establish the diagnosis are also in excess of one million dollars each. Each anesthesia machine is also several hundred thousand dollars. Most patients have EEG and somatosensory evoked potential monitoring to assess the physiology and the neurologic function of the patient while they're asleep during operations to help detect if something is going wrong before it would be too late to correct it. This requires a technician and a neurologist for review and interpretation of these recordings throughout the operation.

All of the surgical instruments and implantable devices and sutures and sterilization equipment have significant expenses, which are added to the prices of the procedures. Behind each one of these medical devices and instruments and pieces of equipment is a company that manufactured it and provides continuous support in the form of personnel for its use and maintenance. Each of these companies has spent years in the research and development of these devices and has a significant amount of monetary investment associated with the development and optimization of these devices. Again, I must reiterate, health care is not free!

It is beyond the scope of this book to discuss in any detail socioeconomic theories such as communism, socialism, and capitalism. Since the advent of the written word and the development of more advanced societies, there has been the realization of social inequalities. There have been the haves and the have-nots seemingly since time began. Kings and emperors are the historical extremes of the haves, whereas serfs and peasants and even slaves have been examples of the have-nots. There have been numerous examples of the masses of have-nots gathering together and toppling regimes of abuse and excess. When those in power controlled the military and had loyalty of the military arm, much bloodshed has been caused by the uprising of the masses. The czars of Russia had incredible wealth but were eventually overtaken by the revolutionaries. The idealism of

Marx was born out of this observation of socioeconomic inequality.

There remains great debate and divisiveness today regarding to what extent the wealth of those who have can be redistributed fairly to those who don't. I have given this little introduction to provoke thoughts about the rationing of health-care expenditures. I don't pretend to have the answer, but simply make the observation that there always has and probably always will be some level of inequality in the world and that includes health care. We have already discussed the problems with government run, top-down regulated health care. It would seem that however well intentioned, all socialistic/communistic attempts at wealth redistribution have not succeeded. Cuba is only ninety miles from Miami, but what a contrast. The Soviet Union has collapsed. China has only flourished as it has adopted capitalistic principles. The current states of Greece, Spain, and even Italy are in severe economic crises due to attempts at wealth redistribution policies. My point is, like it or not, all resources are rationed economically to some extent. Where you live, where your kids go to school, what restaurants you frequent, what you eat, where you shop, what you drive, and where you vacation are all determined by your economic status. As much as we try to deny it or wish it were otherwise, health care is really not intrinsically different and probably cannot be forced to be much different.

The problem today is that hospital bills have become so expensive that the dollar amounts are not realistic and are often inflated and seem excessive compared to the actual intrinsic value. As discussed earlier, hospital bills can have shockingly high charges. Most of the time, the contracted amount that the insurance company actually pays is only a fraction of the charge on the bill. I am not aware of any other field with such crazy accounting practices.

Many have suggested or claimed that medicine is intrinsically different than other parts of the economy and that market forces are generally not applicable as a means of cost controls. I assert that this is a false assumption. There are many clear examples of market-driven cost controls in medicine. It is best seen in the prices of procedures, which are elective and not covered by insurance. Ophthalmologists perform a variety of corneal corrective procedures for patients as an alternative to glasses and contact lenses. When these procedures were new, the costs were high, typically around ten thousand dollars. But now, since many more physicians have been trained in these procedures, they have become much less expensive and are readily available. You can see advertised prices for these procedures for as low as five hundred dollars per eye. Interestingly, it is likely that because these procedures are *not* covered by insurance, that the prices have been driven downward by typical supply-and-demand principles.

If you ever listen to a group of women at a cocktail party when the subject of cosmetic surgery and breast augmentation comes up, it is clear that market forces for these elective procedures are well in play. The women discuss who is performing which procedures and for what price. They seem to know what all the options are for the different sizes and types of materials available. They know which surgical centers are more affordable and which anesthesiologists are both good and affordable. Again, these procedures many years ago were only available to the very rich but now are available to and are utilized by a great number of women in nearly all classes of society.

The knowledge needed to make decisions about which breast implants to choose is really not very different than other health-care choices. The plastic surgeon explains the pros and cons, options and alternatives, and possible risks of the procedure and the patient/health-care consumer makes a choice and decides whether or not the intrinsic value to that person justifies the monetary cost. The doctor, serving as a health-care consultant and service provider, helps the patient to reach a decision for treatment. But it is ultimately the patient who should be responsible for the treatment decision, providing the information and options explained were accurate and appropriate. I sincerely hope that the reader has grasped this subtle but highly important distinction regarding this whole medical economical predicament. The important point is that physicians and health-care providers in general are in a consulting and service industry. Patients come to health-care providers for their expertise and for the services that they offer. Market forces of supply and demand can function in health care as in other industries if this vital distinction is maintained. That is, if people retain responsibility for their health and for how their health-care dollars are spent based on recommendations of health-care providers, then market forces can and should have a significant role in assuring a realistic monetary value of medical services.

Conversely, when responsibility for payments are deferred to insurance companies and the responsibility for the health-care decisions are assumed to be in the hands of the health-care providers and the government, or insurance company, the monetary value for the services are shielded from market pressures, and the monetary values become artificially assigned, and may become completely unrealistic. I believe that we have progressed beyond the era when the doctor was seen as the fatherly figure of Marcus Welby, who simply made the treatment decisions for the patient because the simpleton patient just could not understand the situation enough to make any decision. Today, there is so much information available, literally in the phone in the palm of your hand, that there is very little reason to not be informed about medical options. Physicians, as experienced medical experts, serve as consultants to help people sift through and understand what is and what is not relevant information regarding the condition at hand.

I honestly believe that physicians are at their best when they take the time to educate their patients about their conditions and the options available to them and allow the informed patient to have a role in their treatment. I truly enjoy showing my patients their MRI scans and describing to them why they are having their symptoms and what can and cannot be done to correct their situation. I let them know why I have reached the recommendation I have given and discuss the pros and cons and relative risks of their treatment options with them. If I have done a good job educating the patient and their family, they will be able to be comfortable with either accepting my recommendation or choosing not to. But it is ultimately their choice to make. Doesn't it make sense for you to be the one to make decisions about what happens to your body? The power to choose obviously is accompanied by the responsibility for that choice.

I concede that it may be difficult to apply typical market forces to all aspects of medical care. For example, if you have an emergency situation after a car accident, it is not possible for you to make a negotiation of payment with your neurosurgeon if you are unconscious and require an emergency craniotomy for hematoma evacuation. However, even in this scenario, there can be appropriate pricing guidelines for emergency procedures, which can be regulated by the professionals and insurance companies and government agencies, which are reasonable. For example, if one group of fully qualified trauma surgeons contracts with the hospital they work within to provide emergency services at a certain rate that is lower than a competing group of trauma surgeons, then the group with the lower fees should deserve to obtain that contract unless it is found that the care provided substandard.

It may be difficult in smaller communities to have competitive pricing market forces in play. Oftentimes, there really is only one qualified specialist available, and it is unreasonable for that health-care provider to simply charge whatever he feels he can get away with. I propose that organized physician groups should set standard ranges of acceptable charges for services provided by members of their organizations. This is somewhat different than government regulation but would be hopefully both a realistic and effective solution for some form of cost control. I belong to multiple organized physician societies such as the American Association of Neurological Surgeons, the Arizona State Neurosurgical Society, and the Rocky Mountain Neurosurgical Society. It seems appropriate to me that membership within these accepted medical professional societies could involve an agreement to stay within accepted price ranges, which would be typical and customary for commonly performed procedures. In this way, outliers from the norm could be either banished or otherwise censored from their respective societies. Compensation by insurance companies or government agencies could be contingent upon active membership and participation within appropriate medical professional societies. Currently these societies do not really function in this capacity. These societies are mostly concerned about education and grouping together for some common goals, which are sometimes political in nature. I believe however that physicians could do a better job to police themselves and be more financially transparent by working together on a more economically motivated function through the societies.

I propose that if prices were relatively standardized for common procedures among physician groups, then there would be less of a need for individual contracts and negotiations to be reached between insurance companies and physician groups. Therefore, insurance companies and patients would have more choices available to them for health-care providers and market forces should have a more vital role of cost control, and people would have access to a larger number of physicians. Physicians with good bedside manner and exceptional skills would be obviously more successful within this model, which is what everyone would prefer, rather than insurance companies making contracts with the lowest bidders, unbeknownst to their clients.

THE PROBLEM

I believe that nearly all Americans and most politicians from both major parties actually desire the same thing when speaking of health care. We want good health care, which is affordable. Sounds simple enough, but what does that mean? For most, it means that you have the opportunity to see the physician of your choice in a timely manner when you need to and that you do not have to risk financial bankruptcy when a treatment is necessary. In other words, you should not have to choose between health and financial security. But today, that is what many people face each and every day. The problem today is that health care has become so expensive that it is truly unaffordable for the vast majority of individuals and for the nation as a whole.

In truth, most people don't think about health care at all unless they are sick or have a family member or loved one who is sick. In reality, however, we are all mortal, and eventually, we will all need medical intervention at some time in our lives whether we like it or not. Young people, who are otherwise healthy, almost never consider the consequences of lifestyle choices, such as smoking or drinking excessively, drug use, or risky leisure activities until the consequences of such choices eventually require access to the health-care system. On any given day in our major trauma centers and emergency rooms, there is an endless stream of previously healthy individuals who are now in need of various medical and surgical procedures, which are miraculous on the one side, because of the ability to save lives and restore health to many but which have become extremely expensive. Many young people make a conscious choice to not carry health insurance because of the cost but at the same time decide to purchase recreational vehicles and entertainment systems. Is this responsible?

The most controversial component of Obamacare is the mandate for all people to purchase health insurance in order to address the great burden that the number of uninsured patients in America have on the health-care system. The success of the PPACA clearly depends heavily on this mandate. Without the mandate of every one contributing to insurance, there cannot be guaranteed coverage of preexisting conditions. Anyone should be able to realize that if they were not mandated to pay for the insurance, there would be no need to. They could simply wait until something was wrong with them and apply for insurance after a diagnosis was made since the insurance company could not deny them for any preexisting condition. The controversial Supreme Court decision to uphold this mandate as a tax, even though it was clearly stated not to have been a new tax, remains a hotly debated topic.

The estimates vary somewhat, but approximately forty-five million Americans are uninsured. Much has been written about the potential for the health-care system to be suddenly overwhelmed with new patients if all these people suddenly were covered with insurance. I think this is a major misunderstanding. Every day there are thousands of uninsured patients treated in emergency rooms and in clinics across America. It is illegal to turn someone away in need of care even if they are not citizens of this country. It has been a well-known and longstanding practice to treat these patients regardless of their insurance status. For many, social workers become involved; and if they are eligible, they are placed on Medicaid, and if not, a large bill is generated but is usually never paid. In other words, we already are subsidizing these patients. Unfortunately, however, the conditions may have reached emergency status prior to being addressed and may have been much less burdensome if addressed earlier.

The second major component to the problem is that people do not feel responsible for their health in general or for the cost required to maintain it. The general attitude today is that the government or their insurance company or their employer is responsible. We need to change the mind-set and culture in America to make people realize that they are indeed responsible for their health and for their health care. After someone has reached adulthood, no one else is responsible for that person's, food, shelter, transportation, entertainment, or for their health, other than themselves.

The third component to the problem is that many people feel somehow that health care is a fundamental right, and therefore it should be free. As presented earlier, to assume that something is free is to assume that those who provide the work and service for others would be working as indentured servants or slaves. We must accept that there are incredible individual and corporate and government costs of health care, which do not simply occur without time and effort of many qualified and dedicated individuals, whose service has intrinsic value worthy of compensation.

In the world of Psychology there are well-accepted steps in the grieving process, which occurs in the terminally ill during the dying process and in the survivors after the loss of a loved one. These include Shock, Denial, Anger, Bargaining, Acceptance and finally Resolution. Right now, I believe that most Americans are in the shock, denial and anger phases when it comes to the recognition of the critical illness and eventual death of our current health care non-system. There are very few people who really seem to grasp the extent and reality of the problem as I have attempted to illustrate in the above chapters. In order to begin to fix this very difficult health care economical problem, we must first accept that there is a problem. This problem will not just go away unless there is a fundamental change in the view of health care in America.

First of all, it must be understood that health care is not free. It is not realistic, or affordable for our nation as a whole, to provide the highest level of specialty care and the most modern technological devices, implants and pharmaceuticals for everyone who needs these devices or who could benefit from the use of these items. It would be just as unrealistic to attempt to provide every teenage boy with a Lamborghini who wanted one.

Secondly, we must accept the fact that we are all mortal, and that each and every one of us will die of something, someday, and that it won't necessarily be someone's fault. There are currently many medical problems, which are treatable and even curable, but these treatments can come at a significant expense. You, and only you, are responsible for your life and your health. You are responsible for feeding yourself, clothing yourself, providing shelter for yourself, and for maintaining the health of your body. It costs money to live. It costs money to eat. And yes, it costs money to treat medical illnesses. Your loved ones may certainly wish to assist you in a time of crisis, but it is unrealistic to expect that strangers would feel compelled to pay their hard-earned money so that you can live longer. Again, you are responsible for your life, and if you want to live longer, it is your responsibility to pay for it or arrange to protect yourself from the eventual costs by purchasing health insurance.

If you feel that your life no longer has sufficient quality to keep going, then hospice and comfort care are available. If you feel that although you are currently healthy and in a good state of mind but that you would not want to go through suffering and treatments to maintain a poor quality of life, this fact should be written down and discussed with your loved ones in order to save them difficult decisions on your behalf if you are not able to make them for yourself in the future.

Thirdly, it must be understood that insurance is a means by which many healthy people voluntarily pay a significant amount of their own dollars into a system, which they will never recover, but which should protect them in case they do have a need for access to care in the future. Health care must be understood to be a business within a complex economy. The intrinsic value of the goods and services provided in the medical arena can only be balanced appropriately to other goods and services within the market if free market forces are allowed to function as much as possible. Certainly some form of government regulation is necessary, however top-down regulation and redistribution attempts are far less effective than market pressures in my opinion. In the current situation where health insurance is provided by employers and costs continue to escalate, those costs are causing the companies who provide the insurance to be less competitive relative to other companies overseas. This condition is causing a strain on the overall economy and is costing jobs to be exported overseas. Small businesses cannot afford to provide health insurance to their employees and remain viable businesses. This results in a large number of uninsured people who, when confronted with health conditions, have no means to pay and either become in debt, bankrupt, or dependent on government for assistance, which causes increased national debt and higher taxes for all of us, again putting a strain on the entire economy.

It is an interesting observation that some have made regarding the growth of health care as an industry. Indeed, health care is a recession proof industry and has far outpaced all other aspects of the economy in growth and job development even in this worst of recessions. What is wrong with that? Nothing would be wrong with that if health care was not leeching off all other aspects of the economy for its livelihood. Currently, health care is not a free-standing economic engine but rather a sinkhole and bloodsucker of the vitality of other businesses by consuming increasing percentages of the profits of other businesses in the form of insurance premiums paid by individuals and corporations, and by being a huge consumer of national and state tax dollars.

If you think about it, no one would care if we spent 20 percent of the GNP on automobiles, computers, and cell phones. That is because the production, distribution, sales, and service support of those items supplies jobs and results in tax revenue production. Similarly, no one would be concerned about the amount of money spent on MRI and CT scanners and hospitals *if* the use of these items did not come at the expense of other company's ability to remain viable. Therefore, if people choose to spend their own money on health care due to the intrinsic value to them personally, and health care can stand as a growth industry on its own merits and not primarily as a tax and benefit consumer, no one would complain about how much of the GNP is spent on health care. On the contrary, free market success stories in health care would be applauded in the stock exchange and in the political chambers as job suppliers and tax revenue producers.

When the health care economical problem is discussed in the political arena, it causes great angst on the part of those who feel that their right to health care access will be limited or denied. The huge voting block in the AARP crowd will likely have nothing to do with a candidate or legislative representative who does not promise them to save Medicare. Currently, there is extreme angst on the part of physicians every year when the previously passed law, which called for mandatory cuts in physician reimbursement rears its ugly head. As mentioned earlier, the "doc fix" provision, a stop-gap measure, needs to be voted in each year by congress to prevent a now-required 24 percent Medicare pay cut to physicians. It has increased by about 3 percent per year for the past several years but has never been implemented due to valiant lobbying efforts by physician groups. In fact, if these cuts did take place, it would be very difficult for me to believe that any physicians would take Medicare patients because they would literally be losing money on every patient treated. The current payment levels are so low that many physician groups opt out of taking any Medicare patients already because they feel that they can no longer afford to do so. As the economic wizards have proclaimed, "If you lose money on every patient, you cannot make it up with increasing the volume of patients that you treat.

Physicians are literally torn between feelings of guilt for potentially denying care to patients based on economic factors and the desire to treat all patients in need of their services. The real economic truth is that if a practice goes bankrupt, no patients will be treated. It is a common business analysis of a standard group physician practice to analyze the payer mix. It is considered to be unfavorable for the economic viability of any practice, if a relatively high percentage of Medicare patients are present compared to other insurance providers. In any business other than medicine, it would be standard practice to choose not to do business with an entity, which does not provide adequate compensation for the goods or services provided, which would allow the company to remain solvent. However, because literally human lives and suffering are involved, and there is an uncomfortable necessity of attaching a dollar value to those services provided, things get sticky. Doctors who opt out of Medicare may be viewed as ruthless, cruel, or uncaring and violating the oath of medicine. But what about those in power to make the payment schedules, which place the physicians between a moral rock and an economical hard place? Fortunately for me personally, our business practice specialists have not decided to opt out of Medicare, and I have been spared this moral dilemma. But it has been seriously discussed!

The unfortunate truth is that with the passage of Obamacare, there have been implemented significant additional cuts to the Medicare budget, estimated to be up to the tune of over seven hundred billion dollars. I see no conceivable way that physicians and hospitals can continue to care for Medicare patients with these additional cuts. Even with these cuts, it is projected that Medicare will no longer be solvent within about another decade. Again, the population is aging, and the treatments are more expensive each year. We can no longer put our collective heads in the sand and pretend that this problem will simply go away without some significant changes.

The problem with Medicare and Medicaid, currently, is that they are attempting to provide high-level care for large numbers of individuals, which numbers are increasing daily but with a very limited budget. Many Medicare patients today purchase supplementary insurance as well. Unfortunately, and unbeknownst to most of these individuals, when they purchase supplementary insurance, they often inadvertently subject themselves to many strings attached to the supplementary policies, which actually may limit their choice of physicians and treatment options. There have been many cases in my practice, in which my office staff has informed me, that the patient would have been better off if they were simply on Medicare rather than under the auspices of a supplementary secondary insurance company.

Medicare is a very difficult entity to change or adequately address today because people have paid into the system for many years and rightfully expect to receive the benefit of those payments. However currently, as stated above, Medicare cannot continue to survive as it is currently being implemented. It has become a completely cumbersome government program, uncomfortably melded into the private health-care system without the ability to maintain adequate compensation to health-care providers in the private system for the services required for all individuals older than sixty-five years of age. The demographics of America, with the largest area of demographic growth being that portion of the population over age sixty-five, makes it impossible for the current system to be maintained without major surgery on this method of health-care administration. Medicare rates and rules have become the standard and benchmark from which all other health-care providers are regulated. This has made it extremely difficult for other market forces to take effect.

There is currently a viscous cycle of cost escalation, which is much easier to understand than it is to correct. Let me try to succinctly state the problem and then maybe the solution will be easier to clarify. The pressures favoring escalating costs and utilization of procedures are as follows: Patients present with medical problems for which they feel no personal responsibility in causing. They have insurance, which has mostly been paid for by the government or their employer. The patient feels entitled to have the medical problem diagnosed and treated with minimal or no out of pocket costs. Health-care providers are compensated for performing tests and procedures. The more procedures performed, the higher the compensation. If a diagnosis is missed, or a less than desired outcome is realized, the health-care provider is responsible and may be held liable for not performing a test or a procedure, which may have helped to clarify the diagnosis. There are no financial pressures to restrain tests or procedures. However, there are tremendous pressures to avoid missing a diagnosis, and there are financial incentives to order tests and perform procedures. Therefore all these factors lead to cost escalation. Insurance companies attempt to restrict and limit the ordering of procedures; however, these top-down pressures are essentially ineffective due to the viscous cycle described above. It is my opinion that costs will never decline unless there is a fundamental change in this structure of responsibility. If patients felt personally responsible for their health and health-care costs, things would be different. If physicians were incentivized to consider costs and were freed from severe liability pressures, things would be different. If true market pressures were allowed to function, as in most other segments of the economy, prices would actually respond to those market pressures.

The government has not accepted the problem of care for the illegal immigrants. The Emergency Medical Treatment and Active Labor Act (EMTALA) is a law which prohibits hospitals from sending away anyone in need of medical attention or transferring them to another facility if they have no means to pay for their care even if they are undocumented. The government, however, has not accepted the financial responsibility for these patients. Once someone is admitted to the hospital, it is nearly impossible to discharge them without completing their treatment whether or not they will ever have the means to pay for it. This becomes incredibly difficult when dealing with undocumented individuals.

I was involved in one such case, which resulted in several hundred thousand dollars of unpaid bills for the hospital. This was a tragic situation involving a desperate young brother and sister in their early twenties who decided to flee to America from Guatemala. They had been transported illegally across the border into Arizona by Coyotes (local slang term for those criminals involved in the illegal human trafficking trade). There were reportedly over twenty people crammed into a van, which overturned in the desert while attempting to flee from border patrol agents. All of the passengers were ejected from the vehicle and many were severely injured. Trauma centers throughout Phoenix and Tucson were the final destination for these injured undocumented aliens. I was on neurosurgery trauma call on the night that this young man came in with a broken neck. He was quadriplegic and required emergent cervical spine stabilization and reconstruction. He spoke no English and had only his sister at his bedside to communicate with. Fortunately, she was less severely injured. He remained on a ventilator and in the intensive care unit for weeks until he finally received a tracheotomy and feeding tube and was able to be advanced onto the intermediate care floor where he stayed for months receiving physical and occupational and pulmonary therapies. His sister had no place to live or to go, so she slept in his room at his bedside. Ultimately, the hospital arranged for and paid for a plane ticket back to Guatemala since it was cheaper to provide this transportation than it would be to care for him indefinitely. This is a tragic story, and I felt so badly for this young man and his sister. I can feel good about the care he was given. But the cost was exceptionally high.

Some have suggested that these hospital bills should be simply given to the Federal Government, because they are the ones who have not secured our borders and allow such incidences to occur. But this will likely never happen. The hospital is simply expected to eat the costs since it is the EMTALA law which prohibits hospitals from refusing to care for such individuals. This is an extreme example of a mandate without funding. If there were standard government hospitals and facilities, they would be able to accept these patients and provide further care. Possibly, if the government had more direct involvement in the care of individuals like this case to assume responsibility for, they might feel more strongly about securing the borders.

IF I WERE KING?

Actually, the last thing I would like to be is a king or the president. I just really like being a doctor. But out of frustration at our current nonsystem, and what I view as an absolutely unsustainable and mistaken attempt to correct it, I have written this book in order to inform you, the reader, of the very difficult problem that we are facing. But if I were to become the president and was able to convince Congress to pass meaningful legislation to correct this problem, this is my opinion about what the correct prescription would be.

I honestly think that there needs to be a bona fide two-tier health-care system in the United States, somewhat similar to the situation in Australia. The government should be able to establish a basic level of care to be offered for all citizens who fall below a certain, to be determined, income level. This would be especially helpful for pediatrics and low income/underprivileged families and undocumented citizens, unless the immigration problem is better addressed, and for the elderly with minimal resources. I am not certain that this would require government-built-and-owned hospitals and clinical facilities. However, it would likely best be administered with some infrastructure separate from the private system. Of course, some of these facilities already exist in the form of county hospitals and VA medical centers. Arizona also has an established Indian Health Services system of clinics and hospitals, which are operated through the public health service.

I think it would be quite difficult to administer one basic level of care for some patients and also provide a more service-oriented and higher level of care to other patients right next to each other within the same institution, but with some modifications, that may be possible. It might require the remodeling of some floors within currently existing private hospitals to be separated from and designed for a more basic level of care in one wing and high-end care in another. It also may be possible for private entities to administer government-sponsored health care under a contract to provide for basic level care to underprivileged populations. The renewal of these contracts would obviously be dependent on cost efficiency and quality metrics.

It must be understood that this government-provided care is very basic and limited in its scope and mission. It must be broad-based enough to act as a health-care safety net but not overtake the entire health-care system. All pharmaceuticals and pieces of medical equipment would be generic in nature and available at costs below the private market due to the high volume and nonprofit status. Physicians working in this environment would receive modest compensation compared to private sector physicians but would be completely shielded and protected from any malpractice litigation unless grossly negligent or abusive. Some private physicians may consider an offer to donate their time or work for lower wages as a means of a tax-deductible service for part of their time in these government facilities. This could be one day per week or one week per month for these services. Exceptional and well-known physicians could serve as mentors to doctors in training in these facilities or assigned wards. There could be remarkable opportunities for medical students, residents, and nursing students to work in these clinics and designated hospital wards with supervised autonomy. Some physicians may agree to use that time working in this government system for a certain number of years as a means of repayment for government sponsored student loans.

As part of my general surgical internship, I spent many months working in the VA medical center and in the Phoenix Indian Medical Center. I look back and realize how beneficial this part of my training was in allowing me to perform in more of a primary care role with significant responsibility compared to a more observational role in private hospitals. I was quite humbled to realize that when I was on call at the Indian hospital; I was the point person for all surgical emergencies and consultations for all eleven reservations in the entire state. I will never forget one night when a man was stabbed in the chest and had blood filling up around his lungs causing him to suffocate. I had to evaluate him and determine that a chest tube needed to be placed emergently to save his life. I placed the chest tube and ordered several units of blood to be transfused. Fortunately, his life was saved, and I gained the confidence of knowing that my previously learned medical knowledge had very real needs and practical applications.

Some people with the means to pay for higher levels of care may opt to be treated within the public system, but at a fee commensurate to their financial status, but this would still likely be less expensive compared to that in the private sector. The amount of personal funds expended for this public offered health care would depend on their personal income, up to a maximum rate of 100 percent of the care charges for those who can afford it. Because people would always have this fail-safe backup plan, it would promote a certain level of competition among private insurance providers to maintain a more exceptional level of care with an intrinsic value worth the increased cost. Those patients who have the means to choose whatever care they want, but choose to pay for the government-sponsored care, would help to subsidize the cost of this care for the indigent.

Some would argue that we already have a two-tier system in America with Medicare and Medicaid being provided by the government and private insurance for those who can't afford it. In some sense this is true, but it really does not function in the same way that two-tier systems function and other countries. The problem with the current system is that public dollars are utilized for and attempt to pay for the same level of care as those in the private system. Most of the time, when I'm working in the hospital, I have no idea what insurance plan, be it public or private, the patient is being treated under.

In fact, I have prided myself for choosing not to look at the hospital face sheets when I am asked to consult on any patient so that their insurance status would not sway my opinion for their care even subconsciously.

I have attempted to remain aloof to economic influences in making treatment recommendations for my entire career, assuming that doing what is right for the patient medically should always supersede economic factors. I still believe this is an admirable goal, but it is probably economically irresponsible and unrealistic. Many times, after the fact, I have come to the realization that I have treated someone with an incredibly expensive technology or implantable device and later found that they had no insurance, be it public or private, to pay for such a procedure. This has resulted in a large debt for the patient, which they obviously will never be able to repay. Therefore, the hospital has had to eat a considerable cost because of my generosity. In the past, such generous medical service was possible secondary to higher profit margins and reimbursement rates and higher percentages of insured patients. However, today, the margins are very tight and such losses result in a lack of ability to treat other patients or update necessary equipment.

I have discussed earlier one of the basic problems of attempting to provide the same level of care no matter who pays for the care. This is of course the problem of medical liability. Again to reiterate, it seems inappropriate for people who have no personal financial skin in the game to be able to sue for care that they deem unacceptable. There is a definite perception that all patients are held to the same standard of care from a legal standpoint no matter what their financial situation is after being admitted to the hospital. This doesn't sound so bad, but it is impossible to continue given the economical constraints of our current situation.

I believe that cost savings can only occur when patients themselves are responsible for the care they receive, including financial responsibility. If a patient refuses to make financial arrangements for the care they receive, then they are indeed refusing care. If someone refuses care, they are responsible for the consequences of that choice. I would like to believe that for those people who are truly indigent and incapable of being financial responsible for themselves, the government could step in and be of assistance in providing basic level care under a government-run system. However, those who abuse the good-natured generosity of others cannot simply game the system. A government-sponsored basic level of care, available to all qualified individuals, should ease significant financial burdens of hospitals and health-care systems who are currently subsidizing care in a "mandate without funding" situation. The ability to transfer care to government facilities and make patients personally responsible for their health care can only happen if the legal noose of litigation threats and unfunded mandates of the government are released from the necks of health-care providers.

Care within the government system could reach relatively high levels of complexity and specialization if, and only if, it remained financially feasible. Specialty hospitals could be developed for certain conditions, which may be relatively rare on a local basis, but with significant numbers on a national basis. Alternatively, for rare or exceptional cases, after approved by appropriate medical experts, higher levels of specialty care, only available at certain private centers could occasionally be paid for by the government system as reviewed on a case-by-case basis. Expensive and sophisticated treatments would, for the most part, be avoided due to cost unless proven to be cost effective in the long run, such as epilepsy surgery, and would only be approved for patients after review by a specialty medical board with expertise regarding the condition in question. Cancer treatments, especially those with unproven or minimal utility and high expense, would need to be limited. Prolonged or extended vegetative and custodial care would in general not be supported or maintained at public expense.

Electronic medical records would be kept on all patients in the government system and would allow for national database tracking of conditions and treatments. This would allow for significant improvements in public health administration and clinical research. It should be noted that several smaller countries with nationalized health systems and databases, such as Finland, have provided remarkable epidemiological and long-term treatment outcome data. All people treated within the public health system would have to agree for this type of record-keeping and national database research.

Private sector hospitals would function much as they do now but in a more free market competitive environment. Costs and charges for treatment would be transparent. Insurance companies would need to state clearly and explicitly to clients what is and what is not covered for patients on their plans. People would have the right to personally choose from any number of health insurance policies. Insurance policies would be transportable across state lines and without hidden contractual agreements from certain hospital or physician groups. Patients would be able to choose their physicians and the hospitals in which they are treated, no matter what city or state they reside in. This promotes the development of centers of excellence and cost competitive strategies among institutions providing care. Preexisting conditions would be covered, but may result in higher premiums, up to a predetermined maximum amount as regulated by the government. People in excellent health, who are nonsmokers and physically active with normal body weight, would receive appropriate discounts for their insurance due to their lower risk of illness. This would promote personal responsibility for maintaining optimal health and should result in an overall decrease in health-care expenditures over time.

Insurance would be marketed directly to the consumer rather than being employer based. Companies may still offer health benefits as a means of maintaining an attraction for the best employees and may receive some corporate tax deduction for doing so. However, there would be the same tax deduction available for individuals should they elect to purchase health care on their own. I envision insurance companies competing for individuals in the health-care insurance market in a similar way that car and life insurance companies compete for individual policies today. What is covered on health insurance would be offered in an open and transparent menu like system with each check to an item resulting in an appropriate additional fee. For example, whether or not artificial knee or hip implants would be covered would be a personal choice. This choice would obviously be chosen by the more elderly crowd but could be avoided by young families as a means of diminishing their health-care insurance costs.

On a somewhat more radical note, some people could choose ahead of time to not have cancer treatments included in their plan in order to have their plans be much less expensive. These people would agree to hospice-related comfort care should they be diagnosed with cancer in order to avoid the possible costs of expensive and prolonged cancer treatments should they acquire such a disease at an older age. I think such a treatment policy would be quite attractive to those patients already in their seventies. This is because almost all cancer treatments beyond the age of seventy are rarely curative in spite of being very expensive. However, a young person may be able to include cancer treatments on his or her plan without significant additional expense because the likelihood of contracting cancer is quite low and the possibility of a good outcome with cancer therapy is higher. This would be especially important for women of a relatively young age group who are at some risk for developing breast cancer. Breast cancer today, when detected early, actually has a good prognosis for all but the most aggressive subtypes in most women.

I think most people would choose to have some coverage for all possible infirmities should they contract them but that they may have the ability to choose a maximum dollar amount available for the treatment of these diseases. This is similar to picking the level of coverage on car insurance. Some people may choose a high deductible and relatively low maximum dollar expenditure number in order to decrease their insurance costs. It is obviously impossible to predict what the costs of treatments may be. However, market forces tend to result in conformity and cost adjustments based on what is available. It would be reasonable to have cancer policies with a maximal expenditure of two hundred thousand to five hundred thousand dollars. This amount of money would certainly pay for almost any conceivable upfront treatment plan of care and even most follow-up care. It is well-known that almost all long-term cancer survivors are those who receive the best possible upfront therapy at the time of their first diagnosis. It is quite rare to have salvage therapy after widespread disease has occurred to be successful in the long run. So the strategy would allow for peace of mind knowing that cancer could be treated if detected.

Maximum dollar capitation agreements would also allow insurance companies to more accurately predict their exposure risk and appropriately diminish health-care premiums commensurate to these limitations.

If many people opt out of cancer treatments due to the high expense of treatment, this may actually promote lower costs of these cancer treatments in the future. Furthermore, budget limitations of cancer treatments may result in cancer treatment strategies and products, which are more marketable and available within these cost limitations. Currently, pharmaceutical companies seem to view these cancer drugs that they are developing as being immune to market pressures as if they were given a blank check by insurance companies. I believe that this kind of market pressure over time with transparent and menu-driven personal choice can help curtail the costs of health care in America.

Personal health savings account (HSA) plans are already a very viable insurance product. If people start a health savings plan at a young age and are able to direct their health-care expenditures, significant dollar amounts can accumulate over the years to protect them from significant health-care costs should a serious illness arise. Costs of health care would go down with more people insured in such a system because people would be personally involved and be able to make decisions regarding how and when they spend their health-care dollars. These market forces would curtail costs and promote healthy competition among health-care providers.

One of my associates informed me that after his family became enrolled in a health savings plan promoted by our office, he actually became quite involved in treatment decisions for his own family. He became aware of the variable costs of MRI scans of equal quality offered at different imaging centers. He was shocked to find out that the same MRI scan, performed on the same quality machine and read by the same radiology group could vary in cost from $600 to $2,500. It should be fairly obvious that if people are not forced to go to one imaging center by their insurance plan but are free to choose how their own health-care dollars are spent, the vast majority of people will choose the $600 scans over the $2,500 scans and the more expensive imaging centers will either go out of business or drop their prices.

There are some problems with HSAs and other plans that have a high deductible. It is certainly attractive and results in lower insurance premiums to have a high deductible before any insurance funds are expended. However, this may be a significant deterrent for some people to seek out care when symptoms arise, and this may lead to a delay in diagnoses. Another problem is that people tend have problems in paying there deductible amount, especially if it is a high deductible like a five-thousand-dollar charge. Many times, especially if the physician charge is included in that deductible amount, people simply do not pay the money. I've spoken with some other specialists who have noted this to be a severe problem in their offices. I have been told that people on a payment system will pay as little as five dollars per month on a five-thousand-dollar bill. This is clearly unacceptable and would cause this entire system to be unsustainable if a significant portion of people chose to not be responsible for their deductible amounts. One solution to this problem could be having a modest deductible per incident charge such as a three hundred to five hundred dollar deductible per occurrence while maintaining a total five thousand dollars deductible for the year. This way no single incident would be cost prohibitive and no large debt would be incurred by a single health-care provider. The best health savings accounts, like the one available to our office employees, when fully funded, have the entire deductable amount available for use, but its use is determined by the patient-employee. This means that the costs of office co-pays and deductibles do not come out of the patient's personal pocketbook but out of the funded HSA. But the funds are expended under the personal direction of the patient, so that cost decisions, and thus market forces, are still very much in play for how those dollars are spent.

I propose that large groups of mutually self-insured people, as described earlier, utilizing the type of health savings plans as described above would be the ideal option for many individuals and families. These types of self-insured mutual groups, with elected administrators and transparent administration fees, would be able to offer significant advantages and insurance savings over traditional corporate insurance. I envision large groups of people with the ability to decide for themselves as collective groups what is and is not covered on their insurance plans. Various deductibles and capitated payment expenditures would be available as a choice with payment scales relative to the level of options chosen. The financial health status of the collective mutually self-insured group would be constantly available and transparent on an Internet website for all members of the collective group to see. Voting rights for major expenditures and investments of the group as a whole would be maintained by all paid-up members in good standing within the group. It may be advisable for such groups to have rotating elected administrators in order to avoid any single individual obtaining too much power over the financial decisions. I am involved in many medical societies with such bylaws and rotating elected officials, which function in this type of arrangement, and it seems to work very well. Insurance premiums, which are paid into such collective self-insured groups, would be tax deductible for most people since this would save the government substantial money from the government-provided health-care system and help to incentivize people to be privately insured.

I believe that the current state of Medicare and Medicaid are not sustainable and therefore require a major reform. It seems that a more complete government run health-care system as described above could replace all the basic needs of the elderly and the disabled. Those within the elderly group, who have financial means would be better served by purchasing insurance privately, hopefully with low-cost options and some supplementation paid back to them by the government, recognizing all that they had contributed over their lifetime into the Medicare program. I am also certain that those individuals in retirement, or nearing retirement, may have misgivings about being cared for in a streamlined and basic public health system rather than the current situation, in which they generally can choose the doctor and hospital they want. Again, I must reiterate that the public health system that I envision is not a takeover of the health-care system in America. Those retirees with any means at all could use the dollars, which would be allocated to them for the public system and apply those funds in addition to some additional funds of their own to have full insurance coverage in the private market. Those who cannot afford even the least expensive private insurance plans would have to be content with the public system.

I will admit that the prospect of a full-fledged government health-care system makes the conservative in me nervous. Given the track record of the CBO and the tendency for underestimating costs, there certainly has to be angst among conservatives as a group regarding the prospect of a true national health-care system. There would need to be absolute budgetary transparency and honesty in this system, and mechanisms would need to be in place to avoid going beyond the budget. I also feel that it is extremely important that the people who work within the public health system are incentivized to work and to be rewarded for compassionate care as well as for innovations within the system that result in cost savings and efficiency.

It is also certain that a fully functional public health system would not be put in place overnight. The realization of public clinics and hospital facilities in all communities throughout the nation could be an ultimate goal for fifty years from now, but what about now and the near future of five to ten years? America has a long history of innovation and problem solving. There may be innovative means of tackling this problem. Privatization and contracting for public services has been a means of allowing for innovations in many seemingly nonprivate industries, like prison management, for example. I am really not in a position to judge if this has been successful or not, and I am sure there are critics in this regard, but I am simply making a suggestion of the possibility of alternative solutions.

Although I was somewhat critical of HMOs in my previous chapters, I failed to mention that there has been at least one exceptional example of a large HMO, which has succeeded in providing good care and containing costs. I am speaking of the Kaiser system in California. I have never worked within that system and am certainly no expert when it comes to their type of management and health-care delivery. However, Kaiser, the largest nonprofit health-care system with an enrollment of nearly nine million members, has been held up as an example of a fully integrated care system that has generally succeeded in maintaining a balance of cost and quality. It therefore may be possible for the US government to contact with Kaiser or other similar institutions for developing and managing a more basic but fully integrated public health-care system nationwide. It is interesting to note that the total annual revenue for Kaiser in 2011 was $47.9 billion. If you extrapolate and project coverage for forty-five million uninsured Americans, equaling five times the current Kaiser enrollment, 5 × $47.9 billion equals $240 billion, which is less than half of the current government expenditure of over five hundred billion for Medicare serving a similar number of over forty million Medicare enrollees.

Maybe a public supported but privately administered Kaiser-like approach is the answer.

There are currently some new innovative developments in models of health-care delivery, which are worthy of a brief discussion. *Concierge medicine* is a descriptive term of a type of medical care in which a physician takes a prepaid approach for a defined number of private patient-clients. Each patient-client pays an upfront, monthly dues type of fee in exchange for unlimited 24/7 access to his or her private physician's services. Phone calls, impromptu appointments, and even house calls may be included and agreed upon as part of the services provided and contractually agreed upon. The private physician would come to know each of his or her clients intimately, and a significant trusting and bonding relationship would ideally be established. Obviously, the primary physician would not be a specialist but would be able to address most needs personally and promptly and avoid emergency room visits and excessive tests due to patient familiarity and frequent wellness checks and preventative care measures. Part of the monthly premiums would be applied to a catastrophic care policy for specialty care and/or hospitalization should the need arise. The success of such programs has been dependent upon the primary doctor being adequately compensated for a limited number of patients so that each patient feels that the time allotted for appointments and calls is optimized and the physician is not overwhelmed. Doctors and patients in such models of care delivery have reported high levels of satisfaction and have commented on an improved perception of the doctor-patient relationship.

Another recent development has been in the area of *telemedicine*. In its simplest form, patients call a number and speak directly with a board certified physician for a flat fee. The patient describes symptoms and concerns and receives medical advice and even prescription medications without a doctor visit or examination. In some more advanced scenarios, a webcam on a laptop or iPad can be used for the doctor to visually examine the patient and ask for some routine functions to be observed like walking. Telemedicine avoids the hassle and expense of patient transport to and from the office and certainly is more convenient for simple treatment decisions. Telemedicine used between physicians for consultation, including video and diagnostic imaging sharing capabilities can save significant time and travel costs and can allow subspecialists to consult on a significantly higher number of prospective patients in a very efficient manner. Telemedicine offers the possibility of access to centers of excellence in major cities by individuals in rural and underserved locals at significant cost savings. The potential for missed diagnosis is obvious without direct patient contact but should be relatively rare. However, innovations like telemedicine can only remain successful and viable if provisos for protection against malpractice lawsuits are in effect.

SUMMARY

America became the focal point of medical innovation and education in the early twentieth century primarily because of the opportunities for scientific and medical developments afforded by our free society. Throughout the past one hundred years, medical procedures and equipment have become extremely complex compared to relatively simplistic treatments available prior to the modern era. The development of insurance was initially conceived as a means of making medical treatments more accessible and affordable for the average person. However, with the advent of employer-provided insurance, there has gradually developed a significant confusion regarding who is responsible for one's health and health-care expenditures. Third-party payers have contributed to a complete disconnection of personal financial responsibility for health-care costs and have resulted in uncontrolled cost escalation.

Lawsuit abuse and medical malpractice claims, with often exorbitant lottery-type awards, have resulted in the common practice of defensive medicine by essentially all physicians. Physicians protect themselves from liability by performing numerous tests and procedures, which may be unnecessary if common sense were the driving force rather than the current defensive climate. Ironically, the practice of defensive medicine may ultimately cause more harm than good and certainly has resulted in excessive costs. The costs of medical devices and pharmaceuticals have also escalated almost exponentially because of the inclusion of product liability into the costs of these items. The vicious cycle of cost escalation continues because those responsible for paying the bills are not responsible for the liability and those who desire the treatments are not responsible for paying the bills. Insurance companies have attempted to control costs by increasingly complex regulations and control mechanisms, which make the practice of medicine more frustrating and more costly to administer due to documentation requirements.

Medicare was introduced as a means of providing health care for the elderly; however, this has resulted in a very complex government program with ramifications for all insurance companies regarding standard of care and payment practices. The demographics of America with the baby boom generation now representing the largest subgroup of the population entering and comprising the age of Medicare coverage represents a major challenge for the nation as a whole economically. It is only natural that most medical cost expenditures occur as one gets older and eventually becomes afflicted with a life-threatening process or terminal illness. Unfortunately, all of us are mortal and must face the reality of end-of-life health-care costs. It is not reasonable for public funds to provide expensive and prolonged care for all elderly individuals, especially if the care is futile, or of minimal benefit, in addition to being very costly. When individuals or families are faced with financial responsibility of medical procedures, especially those that are futile, alternative solutions are more likely to be found compared to expensive treatments and procedures.

Medicaid with many different forms, which vary from state to state, is subsidized by both state and federal taxes to assist in the care of the underprivileged. Nearly every state faces significant economical challenges dealing with these health-care expenditures. There are currently approximately forty million Americans who are uninsured. These patients are all currently being treated, in part due to a federal mandate to do so, but in an inefficient and expensive manner, frequently through the emergency rooms of large inner city hospitals. In the past, with fewer uninsured patients and higher reimbursement rates from insured patients, there were enough funds to absorb these nonpaying patients. However, currently, the higher numbers of nonpaying patients and the lower reimbursement rates of insured patients have resulted in severe challenges for traditional hospitals.

Medical-legal pressures force the same level of care to be provided for all patients regardless of a lack of payment for services rendered. Physicians expose themselves to significant medical liability without any promise of compensation by caring for these uninsured patients. This problem has resulted in the outflow of the most economically productive physicians along with their insured patients to specialized surgical centers. If this trend continues, many large city hospitals will no longer be financially solvent and many are already in such a state.

Obamacare, is in my opinion, a flawed attempt at addressing the health-care crisis in America because it attempts to control health care from a top-down regulatory process, but fails to address any of the underlying causes of cost escalation including a complete absence of addressing medical liability. Furthermore, it adds numerous additional taxes and bureaucratic policies and agencies with additional layers of administrative costs and regulations. Ironically, most of the funding sources of Obamacare come from the health-care industry and insurance, which can only increase the cost of private health care for consumers. The other major source of funds for the PPACA is from Medicare, which cannot afford to donate anything to another program and stay functional. Figuratively speaking, Obamacare robs from both Peter and Mary to pay Paul.

The solution to this severe medical economic crisis will require a significant and fundamental change in the philosophy and practice of health care in America. The first and most significant fundamental change among Americans must be an acceptance of personal responsibility for one's health and health-care costs. There has to be an understanding that health care is not free and that the services provided by health-care professionals and the health-care industry as a whole have a significant intrinsic value worthy of just compensation. It is just as unreasonable to assume that someone else would pay for your food and shelter as it is to assume that someone else should pay for your health care. By assuming responsibility for health-care expenditures, free market forces can play a vital role in cost containment and normalize prices of health-care services relative to their real intrinsic value in the market place.

Secondly, it is vital for all of us to accept our own mortality and to come to the realization that when somebody dies, it is typically a result of natural or self-inflicted causes and usually not a doctor's fault. Medical malpractice and lawsuit abuse have contributed immeasurably to the escalation of health-care costs in America. It will never be possible to control health-care costs in America without addressing medical malpractice lawsuit abuse in a very substantial and permanent way. Without the real or perceived threat of litigation, physicians can practice medicine utilizing compassion, common sense, and years of gained knowledge and experience, rather than with knee-jerk defensive tests and procedures.

Thirdly, health insurance must be seen as protection against possible future catastrophic illnesses rather than prepaid health-care dollars to be expended. It must be understood that by paying into an insurance plan, the collective pool of healthy people paying into the system allows for the care of the unfortunate patient when that need arises. People must understand that by paying in small increments over time, the protection provided can give piece of mind for a possible future need but that piece of mind comes at a cost that cannot typically be recovered. People should have many choices about their insurance coverage and be able to choose plans most appropriate to their needs and life situations. I believe that like-minded large pools of people could form and administer self-insured groups, which would be much more cost conscious and equitable compared to large for-profit insurance corporations whose primary goal is to handout large checks to CEOs and stockholders.

Although employers may assist in providing health insurance for their employees, the responsibility for insurance rests with each individual. The insurance market should be competitive for the individual and reflect individual choice so that market forces can play a role in cost containment and product development for the service of the individuals.

Finally, government, meaning the collective pool of all citizens of this country, should be compassionate and conscientious in caring for the poor, underprivileged, disabled, and infirm. However, the government should not and cannot take over the entire health-care system or effectively compete with the private health care. The private, entrepreneur-driven free market medical environment in America resulted in the greatest medical developments in the history of the world, and this environment should be maintained as much as possible.

Private health care must be able to stand on its own merits in a free market, service-oriented environment with cost containment occurring by traditional market forces as much as possible. The government's role in health care should be to provide care to those, and only those people, who aren't able to be responsible to care for themselves. We must accept the fact that government-provided health care will not be equal to or even competitive with the level of care provided in the private system. The government system should be a basic, safety-net level of care designed to provide basic level service and not to attempt to provide full service, modern therapies to all individuals within that system. Those people, who could afford to pay for private insurance, but choose not to, must be held responsible for that decision and either accept to pay for basic level care in the public system or pay for more expensive care in the private system. Since those who chose not to insure themselves would be treated within the public system, the government should have every right to collect for those services in the form of garnished wages and additional individual taxes. In other words, it's not brain surgery; there is no free lunch! It is really not a mandate to have health insurance; it is simply that, if you don't have insurance, and therefore have no other options than to be treated in the public system, you still have to pay for that care.

All citizens would contribute to the national health-care system in the form of taxes, which would take the place of Medicare and Medicaid payments already made today. Additional individual payments for services in the public system would be charged commensurate to the individual's income level. The fee for service payments by those with higher income would help to subsidize treatments of those who cannot afford it. The national health-care service would only be free to those people who truly have no resources.

Health care within the public system would be quite different than health care in the private system in that there would be a significant role of doctors and nurses and therapists in training. National databases and basic clinical research paradigms would be open and transparent within the system. Professionals, who were granted government-sponsored student loans, could pay back these loans by serving in the public health-care system for a predetermined amount of time. More established physicians could choose to work within the public system in roles as mentors to doctors in training with compensation being paid in the form of tax credits or tax deductions. Public clinics would serve as primary care facilities to many of the current frequent fliers of emergency rooms and greatly improve the long-term follow-up care of these individuals in a much more cost-effective manner. The burden on the inner city hospitals would be greatly diminished and this would help restore the vitality of the traditional hospital.

I am certain that there are many additional ideas, which I have neglected to include in this complex medical economic arena. I am also certain that it will take a considerable amount of time and effort for any of the above suggestions to take effect or to have an influence on our current dilemma. However, I firmly believe that with the principles of personal responsibility, limited medical liability, realistic insurance principles, and limited but effective public health care for the indigent, American can remain at the forefront of medical innovation and development. I assert that by following these principles, the costs of health care for the nation as a whole will diminish, and the prices of health-care services will become more commensurate with their real intrinsic value.

Furthermore, by fundamentally changing these health-care principles, America, its businesses, and the free enterprise system will become much healthier economically as a whole, and it will be able to maintain its role as the preeminent world power for the promotion of democracy and peace and individual liberty for the world.

BIBLIOGRAPHY

Barrett, Paul M. "Supreme Court Supports Obamacare, Bolsters Obama." *BloombergBusinessweek*. Retrieved June 30, 2012.

Bliss, Michael. *Harvey Cushing: A life in Surgery*. New York, NY: Oxford University Press, 2007.

Blumberg SJ, Foster EB, Frasier AM, et al. *Design and operation of the National Survey of Children's Health*, 2007. National Center for Health Statistics. Vital Health Stat 1(55). 2012.

Cushing, Lincoln. "Thriving with 1960s-launched KFOG radio – then and now." April 30, 2013, www.kaiserpermanentehistory.org/.

Doyle, Brion B.; Varnum LLP. "Understanding the Impacts of the Patient Protection and Affordable Care Act." *The National Law Review*. Retrieved April 17, 2013.

Feldman, Arthur M. *Understanding Health Care Reform: Bridging the Gap Between Myth and Reality*. CRC Press.

Grier, Peter. "Health care reform bill 101: rules for pre-existing conditions." *The Christian Science Monitor*. Retrieved March, 25, 2010.

Kessler, Daniel P., McClellan, Mark. "Do Doctors Practice Defensive Medicine?" Quarterly Journal of Economics, 1996, v111 (May 2), 353-390.

Leonhardt, David. "Medical Malpractice System Breeds More Waste." *New York Times*, September 22, 2009.

McClellan, JM. "Why New Airplane Prices Are So High." Sport Aviation, January 9, 2013.

McNamara, Kristen. "What Health Overhaul Means for Small Businesses." *The Wall Street Journal.*

Moeller, Philip. "Why You Should Get a Health Savings Account." *US News Money*, May 26, 2013.

Reinhardt, Uwe E. "Changing the Malpractice System." *New York Times*, October 1, 2010.

Slabodkin, Greg. "Problem of Hospital Readmissions, Benefits of Telemedicine Hit Home. *FierceMobileHealthcare.com.*

Vicini, James and Jonathan Stempel. "US Top Court Upholds Health-Care Law in Obama Triumph." Reuters.

Zhou, Katherine. "The History of Medical Insurance in the United States." *The Yale Journal of Medicine and Law.* Vol. VI, Issue 1. November 1, 2009.